After th

After the Change

OLDER WOMEN TALK ABOUT SEX AND RELATIONSHIPS AFTER THE MENOPAUSE

Kathleen Griffin

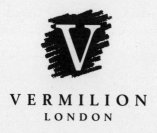

VERMILION

LONDON

First published in the United Kingdom
in 1996 by Vermilion
an imprint of Ebury Press
Random House UK Ltd
Random House
20 Vauxhall Bridge Road
London SW1V 2SA

Random House Australia (Pty) Ltd
20 Alfred Street
Milsons Point Sydney
New South Wales 2016 Australia

Random House New Zealand Limited
18 Poland Road, Glenfield
Auckland 10 New Zealand

Random House South Africa (Pty) Limited
Box 2263 Rosebank 2121 South Africa

Random House UK Limited Reg. No. 954009

1 3 5 7 9 10 8 6 4 2

A CIP catalogue record for this book is available from the
British Library.

ISBN 0 09 181343 3

Printed and bound in Great Britain by
Mackays of Chatham PLC, Chatham, Kent

Papers used by Vermilion are natural, recyclable products made
from wood grown in sustainable forests.

For my mother, Monique, and Gerald, my late father,
who lit the path ahead with their love and encouragement.

Contents

Acknowledgements

Many women helped this book see the light of day. For several years, everyone I interviewed as a journalist, or met socially, was greeted with the same questions about menopause. Most of them must remain anonymous, but they know who they are and they have my heartfelt thanks. The women who agreed to be interviewed for the book were frank and honest, and this is their book as much as mine. Thanks to all who gave time and enthusiasm to discuss the project. Special thanks to Help the Aged and the Amarant Trust.

Maryrose Tarpey gave me invaluable information about qualitative research and kept me going with telephone coffee breaks. Corinne Sweet was always there when I needed her. Thanks also to friends and family who steered me through the stormier waters: Monique Griffin, Tim and Isobel Griffin, Françoise Griffin, Frances Randall, Marilyn Gascon, Paul Milnes, Mary Ambrose, Clarinda Cuppage, Hazel Castell, Lyn Webster Wilde, Tim Salmon, Fiona Hill and Marlena Spieler.

Dermot Maguire and Nick Mann of Barclays Bank gave me financial support when it mattered most.

My agent Jane Judd and editor Hilary Foakes showed patience and encouragement. Lucy MacArthur did research and her administrative support was invaluable in those last frantic weeks.

Thanks to all at Woman's Hour for their support and good humour.

And finally to the masters, Studs Terkel and Tony Parker, who have always been an inspiration.

Introduction

In 1984, I was having strawberries and cream with a friend in north London. Steve Davis, a particular favourite of hers, had just won the World Snooker Championship. We chatted happily about the match and compared previous champions. Suddenly Marie, as I shall call her, turned to me and said, 'Can I ask you something?' I smiled and nodded, assuming that she wanted me to take her out to do a bit of shopping. 'Only I can't ask anyone else.'

'Sure, go ahead.'

'What is sex really like?'

I was astonished. Marie was eighty-five years old, single and a pillar of the Baptist community. 'Only I can't ask any of my other friends – they'd be too shocked and I thought you are the only person I know that I can ask.'

So how do you explain what sex feels like to a virgin in her eighties? I knew that Marie had never married, her fiancé had been killed in the First World War, along with a whole generation of sweethearts, but I'd always assumed she had no interest. Women of her age didn't, did they?

I thought for a bit – how do you explain, after all? Then, taking a deep breath, I said, 'Well, when it's good, it's like . . .' – searching for a metaphor that would do it full justice – 'like the best strawberry ice cream you've ever had.'

Now it was Marie's turn to look astonished. 'That good!' and we both burst into fits of giggles, while I went into more detail.

Later that afternoon, driving home, I was struck by the oddity of a woman in her twenties explaining about sex to a woman who had always been financially independent, and might have been expected to be more 'worldly', and was old enough to be my grandmother. And then, if I was honest, I was more surprised by the fact that she still wanted to know, rather than by her ignorance. That same week, while visiting another friend in her eighties, we got to talking about relationships. Jess had been married twice, unhappily both times. I knew she had survived the Blitz and had brought up her family through all the hardships of the war in the East End. But she had never gone into details about her husbands.

'The first one was the sort of man who would steal your eyeballs and spit in the sockets. I left him. The second one was all right to start with and we had the four kids. He was violent, but so were they all. He was no different from all the neighbours. But I left him one day when he picked up the television and threw it at me. I drew the line at that. I lay awake all night planning my escape. When he went to work the next day, I made him his breakfast as usual. Then when he'd gone, I dressed the kids, packed a case, put my coat on, put the key on the table and left. Never looked back and never saw him again.'

Jess smiled and described the hardships of bringing up four children on her own. Again, I thought that I had never imagined this frail old lady having the courage to walk out on a man, with no money, nowhere to sleep even.

I was a young journalist and filed this under 'interesting story' in my head. Several years went by and then another friend said to me one day, after a dinner with several glasses of wine, when the conversation had turned to relationships and sex, 'Look, I'm seventy-five years old and now I'm ill. I've been thinking, I've never slept with anyone, but I don't want to miss out on the experience before I die. But how does someone my age set about finding someone to sleep with?'

Again I found myself surprised that she should still be so curious, so late in life. And then two days later, another friend who had been happily married for more than fifty years, put down her cup of afternoon tea and said, 'Kathleen, there's been something I've been meaning to ask you, I hope you don't mind?' I looked at the lawn, which needed a good trim and was preparing to get up and go down to the shed at the bottom of the garden. 'What's it like to sleep with more than one man? You see, Henry and I, well I'd never known anyone before, and it's lovely with him, but sometimes I do wonder . . .' she giggled nervously.

I gulped, then I remembered Marie and ice cream came to the rescue again. 'Well, you love vanilla ice cream, but sometimes you fancy some pistachio, it's a bit like that, different flavours but equally scrumptious.' And then I did go and cut the lawn. While I was walking up and down, trying to make reasonably straight lines, I wondered how many older women out there still thought about sex at all. Women my age were always comparing notes, but I'd never read any comments by older women. And then I remembered my conversations with Marie and Jess, now both dead.

Women of my generation talked about sex with one another and with men of our own age. It was more difficult to talk with women of our mothers' age. So we tended to assume that they never talked about it, worried about it or laughed about it as we did, let alone had sex themselves. The cut-off point, I had always imagined, was around menopause. So just how did older women feel about their sexuality and how did menopause affect things?

I decided to take menopause as the starting point, because it seemed to raise so many issues of age, fertility, self-image and sexuality. In the same way that the onset of periods is a clear beginning in a woman's life, in the sense that there is a before and after, was menopause the same, but at the other end of a woman's life, a clear ending?

Scanning the shelves of the library, I was struck by the way older women's experiences had been categorised. There were plenty of books about the menopause itself, mostly anthropological tomes of faraway islands or sociological texts. And then there were wheelbarrows full of self-help books; menopause and diet, exercise and menopause, several American books of the 'It made no difference to me, menopause, what menopause?' school. But I couldn't find a single book in which women described their own sexuality at menopause. They were invariably quotes stuck into someone else's theory.

I began talking to all the older women I met through my work as a journalist and floated the idea of a book about older women's sexuality. It was as if I had suddenly become a member of a secret club. 'Of course we fantasise and talk about sex, it's just that your generation think they invented it', 'I wouldn't ever talk about it, but I do wonder', 'My grandmother's been having affairs for years.'

I talked the idea over with my agent, Jane Judd, who was immediately enthusiastic, but felt it must have been done before. Further digging drew a blank and she approached a publisher who had the same reaction.

It seemed vital that older women should be allowed to speak for themselves. As a radio journalist, I was used to conducting interviews, sometimes difficult and intimate ones. But this was different – would women willingly talk to me? I began to ask everyone I met; interviewees, dinner guests, the woman in the corner shop, if they thought women would talk and if they knew anyone I could talk to.

Within weeks I had a first list of a dozen contacts. I went to the large charities; Help the Aged, Age Concern and to the Amarant Trust. Soon I had lists of names and was beginning to ring potential interviewees. I'm good on the phone – I have to be, I ring dozens of people every week to pester them for a comment, a reaction or an interview. But this was different. Ringing up complete strangers, some old enough to be my grandmother, to ask them if they would mind talking to me about their sexuality!

The reaction I got underlined the fact that I was on to something. No one, of the dozens of women I called, slammed the phone down, or told me to mind my own business. After all, how would I feel if someone rang with the same request? If they felt they couldn't help, they'd give me the name of two or three friends who could, or who had interesting stories to tell. It quickly became clear that there was a rich untapped vein of experience here.

I felt it was important to get a cross-section of experience; happily and unhappily married, widowed, celibate, gay. Reading through the available literature, it soon became clear that my sample was not going to be representative unless I interviewed hundreds of women. But I was not doing academic research; what I was after was a patchwork of women's lives for readers to draw their own conclusions.

I read the masters in the field of this type of interview, Studs Terkel and Tony Parker, and realised that what had always touched me about their work was the openness of the interviews, without an underlying theoretical matrix. Of course this went against all sound journalistic training. I wasn't looking for a story, but allowing myself to be a human tape recorder.

Having talked to dozens of women about their experiences, I whittled the numbers down to twenty. I wanted the reader to feel by the end of the book that she or he knew these women and cared about their lives. But I also wanted the reader to understand the different issues involved. I decided to divide the book by chapter headings, rather than by individuals.

Experience of menopause, marriage and long-term relationships, society, fidelity, death, celibacy were all on the original list. When I started interviewing I did so chapter by chapter. It soon became clear that I needed another chapter on men and one on the new generations and that certain topics – death and health – could be included within other chapters.

I wanted to strike a balance between how I saw the shape of the book developing and the patterns that were beginning to emerge from the interviews themselves.

All interviews began with a discussion of the ground rules. Interviews were to be completely confidential with names and identifying details changed and disguised. If at the end of an interview, any woman felt that she had said too much, she was free to withdraw that part of the interview. The recorded interview would not be used for a radio series I was planning without their permission. People speak differently if they know their opinions are not going to be broadcast and we couldn't conduct the interviews using both criteria. I thought that the women might regret their revelations. But for a few small details, no one did. Only two people subsequently withdrew their permission for me to use their interviews. I thank them both for the valuable contribution they made to my awareness of the subject.

It was important to make clear that this was not a book about sex as such. I wasn't interested in details about hanging from the chandeliers, but about sexuality. After all, some of these women would no longer still be having sex, but were still sexual.

My questions would be edited out of the transcriptions and the final interviews would be edited in the normal way, so that the hesitations and repetitions that make verbatim accounts difficult reading, would be edited out. I wanted the accounts to stand very much by themselves, without the interruption of question and answer. In this way, each woman's experience would flow into the next, to create a patchwork of impressions on the subject under discussion.

During the interviews, I allowed myself to be led by the women themselves, which quickly threw up new questions. It was a difficult balancing act between leading and being led, but I needed to follow *them* if I was going to get an accurate picture of their experiences, rather than what I thought their experiences should be.

Most women seemed to go through menopause in their late forties and early fifties. But I was keen to interview a spread of women, from those who had just gone through menopause, to women in their eighties. And what about women who had had a hysterectomy and so had an early menopause?

Eighty year olds would have experienced other factors that would have influenced their lives; world wars, the depression. And they would have been brought up by a different generation again, the Victorians. I would be talking to several generations of women. How had they been brought up, informed about sex? Had they led sexual lives before marriage, and how had this affected their views? And how had they raised and informed their own children? How did gay women feel about long-term relationships, were their experiences any different? What was it like being gay at their age?

I then wanted to write a conclusion, drawing together

some of the ideas expressed by the women in the book. I have also added a cast list that the reader can refer to in order to remember details about each woman. The cast list also has page cross references, so that if the reader becomes interested in a particular woman, she can follow her story through the book.

I was not prepared for the frankness and enthusiasm of the women I interviewed. With a complete stranger, they were delighted to plunge into the most intimate details of their lives. At several points during the interviews, I found myself wondering if I would have been as frank about my own life. That was the first surprise – these women had been waiting to talk, longing to talk, no one had ever asked them what they thought and felt and needed before.

We wouldn't dream of assuming that a woman in her twenties had the same outlook on life as a woman in her fifties, yet society lumps all post-menopausal women together. Yet a fifty year old is as far from an eighty year old in experience as from a twenty year old. I will never be able to look at an older woman in quite the same light again.

Chapter One

The change

Menstruation is our first experience of what being a woman really means. While the adolescent girl may have noticed changes in her body, the onset of periods is a public recognition of her new status. Immediate family and friends will be told and schoolfriends will compare notes as to who has 'come on' and who hasn't yet started. While the status may only yet be dimly perceived by the young woman herself, somehow she realises that this is an important step, partly from the reaction she gets from her immediate circle.

But it is also a time when childish freedoms must be left behind and a new persona assumed. While boys have a clear route through adolescence, periods for girls mark the before and after and there is no going back. Many women I spoke to reported feeling they had left something behind when their periods started, a person that was really them, a person they only re-encountered at menopause.

The menstruating woman is powerful, a symbol of fertility, but that power is also feared. In Turkey, for example, women menstruating are thought to be a threat to social order. Many of the great world religions have ambivalent attitudes to periods; in the past women in different religions had to cleanse themselves ritually after periods to be readmitted to the religious group.

Historically, menstruation announced the beginning of a life that was charted out for the young girl, restricted in a way that a man's life never would be. She would be loved and protected and in return must give up her independence and conform. A husband would be found, she would 'settle down' into marriage and motherhood. Those who did not follow the plan would be ostracised as spinsters. As recently as the nineteenth century, spinsters were wholly dependent on the good will of the rest of the family, the 'surplus women' referred to so disdainfully in fiction, might and did starve. So for the older generation, now in their late seventies and eighties, there simply was no other path. Periods announced a path traced out to the grave.

In more modern times, in the great kitchens of the world, periods were used as an excuse for prejudice. Women were banned from the professional kitchens of the great restaurants and hotels. Various excuses were put forward – they made mayonnaise curdle, soufflés wouldn't rise, meat would go off more quickly – all laid at the door of periods.

Many other careers were also closed to women; the British navy has long believed that it is somehow unlucky to have women aboard ship, ordination of women priests was met with a flurry of panic by the male establishment, orchestras have only recently begun to welcome professional women musicians. The excuse given was physical weakness or tradition, the fear an ancient one that came from menstruation, the belief that women have some mysterious power that might infect the masculine world.

The history of medicine has encouraged women to believe that a vital part of them is situated in the womb, that it is the centre of their womanhood. In the nineteenth century many people believed that the womb was a live animal which could move around the body. In rural areas of Switzerland, when women had abdominal operations, they used to make little toads in wax and leave them as votive offerings by religious shrines.

The notion of the hysteric goes back to ancient Greece when the woman was defined as being her womb. In the nineteenth century in America, it was thought that a woman could be driven mad by her organs, and hundreds of unnecessary hysterectomies and ovariectomies were done on healthy young women. Folklore held that the womb was somehow full of mysterious powers. Linked to fertility, it could produce life so what else might it not do?

But while the start of periods in teenage years marks the passage from girlhood to woman, menopause is a step in the dark. If women are defined by fertility or the potential to bear children, how is their essential womanliness to be lived when this is taken away? And with women living longer, healthier lives, the older woman is no longer the same person she was a hundred or even fifty years ago.

And however welcome marriage and children are, many women feel they lose their identity; fertility gets in the way, clouds the subject, because life then becomes a busy wheel of catering for husband and children. Simone de Beauvoir in *The Second Sex*, said, 'One is not born, but rather becomes, a woman', and that becoming is shaped by society through the approved routes of marriage and childbirth.

Menopause seems to crystallise a woman's experience; a rocky road often reflects a bumpy passage through life. Menopause frequently coincides with a time when children are leaving home and that underlines the change in role. Yet the sympathy and approval signalled by the beginning of periods disappears. How many jokes do you know about the beginning of periods? And while periods may have been awkward and embarrassing for the teenager caught without tampons, what about the fifty year old in a restaurant who suddenly begins flooding?

The menopausal woman is a laughing stock in the lexicon of comedy in our culture; a figure of fun with her hot flushes, dry vagina and hairy chin, her tendency to shoplift and panic. But because all these things can happen to her, it does not mean they will.

But what role models are there? Which sensible woman volunteers the information that she is menopausal, knowing what the reaction is likely to be? That at the very least she will no longer be taken seriously, that any temporary slip will be put down, with a knowing wink, to the change? The media seems to have two models for the menopausal woman; the monster from the deep and the (generally famous) woman who sails through it all. So she is caught somewhere between the lunatic and Joan Collins.

The plethora of self-help books on diet and exercise serve up the usual menu of guilt offered to women of all ages, but this is refined torture. Eat this diet, do this exercise, swig this magic potion and nothing will happen! Life will go on as before and, most importantly, *no one will know*. It is the same message that women have been receiving throughout life; this is how you can cheat and fool the world into thinking you are still in your late twenties, because that is how the world wants you to be. But judgement is harsh if you should fail and miss the target, four little words that evoke scorn and pity – 'mutton dressed as lamb' – a menacing mantra chanted as you pass, even if only in your own head.

'Passing' for younger is the supreme compliment in a society that assumes no normal woman in her right mind would want to look her age. So we tuck and trim, agonise over wrinkles, trying to halt a process that will happen anyway, however much we kick and fight. While a man's sexual potency may be called into question, his basic ability to attract women, wrinkles and all, grows with age. An older man with a younger woman on his arm is often admired, his sexuality is enhanced, he can still father

her children. But the scorn that often greets an older woman with a 'toy boy' shows how fertility is the base line of approval. By this measure, every menopausal woman is the same, literally useless.

And yet the reality is different. Every woman has her own menopause, as individual as her experience of periods or childbirth. One woman in her eighties complained about being taken to a day centre to play bingo with other people her own age. She would turn off her hearing aid in protest; 'I've never liked bingo, why should I like it now, just because I've turned eighty?' We wouldn't dream of thinking a twenty-year-old woman had the same feelings or enthusiasms as a forty-year-old. Yet we lump everyone past menopause together, from the fifty-four-year-old high flier to the great grandmother in her eighties.

Feminism has allowed us to re-examine our lives as women. The important milestones in our lives – first periods, first sexual encounter, marriage, childbirth etc. – have been given a new significance. Many older women haven't accepted this new analysis. They remain in a political vacuum, unhappy with the way society treated them, but unwilling to accept the feminist perspective and unable to put forward an alternative interpretation. Women in their eighties tend to think that a lot of fuss about nothing is made about menopause, that it is just something to get on with. Their grandmothers were the ones accused of being hysterics by nineteenth-century doctors.

Women in their sixties have refused to suffer as their mothers did, many turning to HRT or having hysterectomies. HRT itself divides women into two camps – disciples and enemies. Many of the women I spoke to swore by the treatment, wanting to remain younger and hoping it would give them protection against osteoporosis. Other women were keen to go it alone, experiencing the change and reluctant to put themselves into the hands of doctors.

The way they experienced menopause also depended on what else was going on in their lives – economic difficulties, marital tensions, problems with children. Mothers who had children in their forties seemed to have an ambivalent menopause; because they were the mothers of young children while going through the change they received different signals from society and generally had an easier passage.

Many women perceived a difference between aging and menopause, seeing the latter as a natural part of life. One woman resisted all the symptoms and evidence of menopause as much as she could, believing that she could fend it off if she pretended it wasn't happening, when she saw all her friends disintegrating around her.

Sex also changed. For some the practical problems of a drying vagina and wrinkles brought dilemmas. Many more women mentioned the new freedom they felt at not having to worry about pregnancy. Some also mentioned a surge in sexual feelings to unknown men, the fancying of younger men on the bus home from work syndrome. Some women were embarking on new relationships, with the same fears and questions of women in their thirties.

This chapter looks at menopause as a way of examining women's sexuality. How much was it a rite of passage? Were women's experiences different from the prevailing literature which seemed to divide menopause into a devastating, depressive illness or 'I can cope with anything' bounciness? Was menopause a time for stock taking? How did it affect other areas of life? Did it change attitudes to sexuality in self and others? How was it different from aging? Had women been able to talk about their experiences with others? Were they able to compare with previous generations, had their mothers told them what to expect? Did HRT, which seemed to cause such controversy between believers and non-believers, really make any difference? Who is emerging at menopause? Could it be the real woman, hidden by a lifetime of serving and being available, however willingly?

Women suddenly felt able, with the alibi of menopause, to behave 'inappropriately'. They got angry, bought themselves that new bright yellow jacket, took a holiday they couldn't afford, refused to go to that dinner party with the people who had been boring them for years. Could this just be a question of hormones?

I was struck time and again how positive women seemed once they had come through menopause, how confident, with a self-assurance that often seems missing in younger women. Society no longer needed them, they could no longer have children. In other times they would have hardly lived more than a few years, so the questions were never asked. But now a woman can be healthy and strong well into her eighties and then she does begin to reflect and ask questions.

And more than anything she has time and space. Time for herself, to dig the garden, go on a course, or just sit and think. Time to speak to her daughters, or more often her granddaughters, and pass on what she has learned. Simone de Beauvoir said, 'Woman is now delivered from the servitude imposed by her female nature. And what is more, she is no longer the prey of overwhelming forces; she is herself, she and her body are one.' Many women I spoke to had the same reaction; they finally felt they had been let off the hook, somehow sneaked back into their own secret garden which they had been forced to leave at puberty.

Marjorie

Seventy-six. She comes to the door in a black leather trouser suit, a tall woman surrounded by her beloved dogs. The coffee is generously laced with brandy. Feisty is the word that comes to mind.

Do you want me to speak frankly? I think the fuss about menopause is a load of balls! People tell you these dreadful stories. Maybe because it didn't happen to me, I'm a bit hard-hearted about it. It's a matter of what you expect – if you don't expect these things, generally speaking they don't happen.

Frankly I don't remember when I went through menopause, I didn't even notice it at the time, I was so goddamn busy. And the obvious symptom with me has always been a matter of come and go, so when it didn't happen I was just quite pleased. I didn't get hot flushes or mood swings, well I may have got bad tempered but I had other reasons for that! I suppose there were other things to make me have hot flushes of rage too, because my marriage was breaking up at that time.

I must have been about fifty-four when I went through menopause. I didn't feel any different. I was just damned glad that I didn't have to worry so much, you know, the other thing was over. There was no one else involved at that time anyway so it didn't really matter. I had had my fill of men. I had reached the conclusion that men were good for one thing only and some of them weren't much good at that either.

Marjorie seemed an odd mixture of reticence and bluntness. She'd be coy about references to sex, and then launch into a tirade about a favourite subject, with swearing that would not have disgraced a building site! She'd recently had a cataract operation and apologised for her puffy face, though she was still wearing 'the full war paint'. Of all the women I interviewed, she surprised me most by her appearance and attitude – she had the mind and opinions of a younger woman in an older woman's body. And it wasn't just the leather trouser suit, but the way she unconsciously swung her hips in a sexy way when she walked. When she took me back to the station with one of her dogs, she drew admiring glances and wolf whistles from passing cars. They were clearly understanding the signals she was giving out – it was hilarious to watch their faces as they came by and realised they had been flirting with a pensioner. Marjorie seemed to float above it all, pretending not to notice. Though her eyesight is none too good, I'm sure she was aware of everything that was going on!

Evelyn

Fifty-six. She has a smoker's cough which comes upon her when she laughs, which she does often. A no-nonsense woman.

It's a milestone, not a big one but something's got to point to death hasn't it? [*She throws back her head and laughs.*] I think we are more conscious of menopause than our mothers were. Most of my friends are round about my own age and are going through it in one way or the other. Some don't speak about it at all, others make a big issue out of it and others are far more accepting of it.

I like to think I have accepted it. I hope that I'm living day to day, passing the time away. A watershed in the aging process from birth to the grave! I suppose it's been a positive experience, salutary.

I rage against whiskers on my chin and the fact that I can't run without getting out of breath, but that may be something to do with being overweight! I haven't got the stamina I had, I can't lift such heavy weights now, I can't go on for so long, I can't eat late at night. Those are the sorts of things I rage against, but that's aging not just the menopause. It's got to be positive hasn't it, because you've got to accept it. You can't do anything about it, you can't reverse it.

Menopause, if it was something that happened, bang like that, might change you more radically, but because it's something that creeps up on you, you're going through the change experience without even realising you're doing it. I mean you're not changing from green to red like traffic lights; it's a slow process.

The youngest of ten children, Evelyn lives right out in the country in the north of England. She seems resigned to her life, accepting what fate throws at her with a grim smile and another fag. She sits with her feet curled up under her on the sofa and pokes the fire to punctuate her most important points; it's the centrepiece of a comfortable sitting room.

I'm puzzled by her reactions to my questions – often she says something cutting or cynical and then throws back her head and laughs, as if gauging my response.

I feel she has had some bitterness in her life, but dug her heels in and got on with it. She enjoys her social work, though is miserable and depressed about a particularly difficult child abuse case she's currently working on.

Rose

Eighty-four. It's a cold day so we sit in the kitchen, the warmest room in the house and drink endless cups of coffee in her sheltered housing flat. She has a warm, old-fashioned way about her.

I was taken bad, to hospital, it was to do with my spine. I had no period during all that time and I was there for six weeks. The nurse said, 'Oh you'll be coming back here in about another eight months.' I didn't know what she meant.

I saw my doctor after about three or four weeks. I had these terrible hot sweats come on, I could not make it out. I was only in my thirties. It was a horrible feeling all these hot sweats. The doctor said you must expect that now you're in your forties, and I said no, I'm still in my thirties. Anyway my mother couldn't make it out, and she got her doctor to examine me and he couldn't make out what was wrong. I went to the medical mission, when we got there I saw a doctor and she examined me and said your ovaries are drying up – and I was thirty-seven. She said, we might be able to force a period. I asked her if she agreed with it and she said she thought it's not natural, anything's not natural I'd rather leave it.

I felt very angry, I'd have loved to have had another child, a girl. I already had one son, just before I was nineteen and then five years later I had another one. It seemed that I was still young and I wanted another child. I felt it's not my time to finish having my periods and I thought to myself it didn't seem fair. I wondered what caused it.

My sister was getting on for fifty when she was finished. It made me feel as if I wasn't really a woman still. It also affected me physically, terribly dry skin, I've had it ever since. These days they're so up on everything, but in those days they didn't realise. I felt old suddenly, I felt like I was in the middle age and yet I was still young.

Everybody says that I don't look my age now. I wonder if it has affected me in the long term – my health has been on and off for many years. I've been in and out of hospital, I've got a plastic artery to the heart and that was thirteen years ago.

It affected my life with my husband. We had trouble when we had intercourse, I used to seem to have a lot of pain. You get very dry but I didn't know none of that then. No one knew anything. My husband's health was poor, so he never used to want to make love with me that much, and for me, it seems as if I turned off. I suppose my body was beginning to feel like the body of a woman about fifty.

Everyone's favourite grandmother, Rose is a warm, affectionate woman who has lived in the same part of the city all her life. She's always had to make do and mend. When she opens the cupboard to get the jar of instant coffee out, there's hardly anything else in there. She manages on her weekly pension.

While she's boiling the kettle and getting the milk and sugar out, we chat about current affairs. She's shocked at the latest government cuts. A lifelong Labour voter, she's recently been active in campaigning for rights for pensioners.

She doesn't complain about her own circumstances, accepting what life brings and grateful for the love and affection of her large extended family, whose photographs are everywhere. I'm appalled that someone who has worked so hard all her life should have so little and yet be so accepting.

Elizabeth

Seventy-seven. She walks with a stick, but has just been admiring her garden. She is smartly dressed with bright blue, mischievous eyes.

Quite honestly I was so busy with my family, because you see I had my last two children when I was in my forties, at forty-one and forty-four, so I really didn't have a lot of time to think about myself. That was probably a very good thing. I had a pretty good menopause, it started when I was about forty-seven.

It was just the natural sequence of events, it didn't worry me in the slightest, I can't honestly think of any real symptoms that I had at all. If I had mood swings, it could have been just when the children got on top of me but I didn't have any of this awful depression. I'm sure it did keep me younger, the main thing was that I had so much to occupy me, so much to think about, I didn't concentrate on myself at all.

For so many women when they get to the menopause, life has rather lost its point, because your children are grown up and possibly you and your husband have drifted rather. Unless you've got a job that you're enjoying, life has become a bit pointless. But you see I was lucky, I had the children to think of all the time and all their varying interests. My eldest son got married when my youngest son was two and I had the rest of them at home. I felt awful when my last son went because I found it very difficult to adjust to being just two of us, particularly with cooking.

I was a mother of young children in my fifties. It was

very unusual among the people I knew. My sister-in-law frowned on it, she was absolutely horrified, very, very disapproving! It wasn't a nice thing to do! Of course she was horrified anyhow that we had so many children because she reckoned that we couldn't afford them, well by present-day standards we possibly couldn't, but we were happy. My really close friends were surprised and quite sympathetic but not disapproving.

It wasn't any more difficult than when I was younger. I enjoyed the last two children more than any of them. I was very upset, at first, when I found out I was expecting the fourth baby, after all I thought I'd finished with children and also I had got a job I was enjoying very much, but once she was born that was it, I was thrilled to death. I really enjoyed her.

Elizabeth is the frailest of all the people I interviewed. She looks as if a puff of wind would blow her over. She has put her whole identity into her life as a wife and mother. She enjoyed her two later pregnancies, as this meant she could prolong motherhood indefinitely. In her fifties she was both a mother of young children and grandmother, a role she clearly revels in. She emphasises the nurturing role and not concentrating on herself, giving herself wholly to the needs of others. She has lived a life that women throughout the ages would recognise. It leaves me wondering what space she has left for herself, though she would probably consider the idea nonsense!

Annie

Fifty-six. She lives in a sunny basement flat full of cats who are petted and fussed over during the interview. She is shy and nervous at first.

I found it and am finding it quite a depressing experience. I'm very happy not to have periods anymore, I don't miss them, some women say they do. I equate menopause with aging. A friend who is a bit older than me was talking about menopause and she said 'Hold on a minute, you're equating menopause with aging.' In my case, it amounts to the same thing, because it was a fairly late menopause.

I had my last period when I was fifty-four, I find it difficult to date. I had hot flushes for a short while, but my periods were very irregular for about two years before that. I rang up my sister who's five years older than me, when my periods started being irregular, and I said 'What happens when you go through menopause?' She's an ex-nurse, and she said, 'Well, it's different for everybody'.

I didn't quite know whether I was getting hot flushes and I wanted to know what was coming next. Basically nothing came next! One thing I did notice, I used to suffer terribly badly from hands and feet going dead and that doesn't happen anymore, so something has happened to me that is making my body warmer.

I rather dreaded it. I remember seeing my mother loosening the clothes round her collar, flapping her hands around her face and fanning herself with all the windows open, and generally getting into a state and this was one of the things that I expected.

I had a very depressing experience the other day. I went to the doctor for a smear. The last one I had was rather painful, three years ago. I put it down to their being perhaps a bit clumsy, but this time the nurse started to do it and the pain was excruciating and I had to ask her to stop. Then she went and got a smaller speculum, the smallest one they can use and she put water on it and I had to stop her again. She went to fetch the doctor, who was really sweet, they were both very nice to me and explained what was happening. Your skin inside dries up, and whereas they weren't telling me anything that I didn't know, I found that profoundly depressing, my body saying to me very clearly you have dried up sexually. And I actually came home and I had a bit of a weep about it. It's symbolic and very, very clear.

Annie was dressed in an old track suit, which she pointed out to me was the only thing she could get into nowadays, and was the one woman I talked to who seemed most unhappy about the way she looked. As a gay woman who has had to hide her sexuality for years, she has been very saddened and depressed by her life, brought on by the unbearable tensions of her hidden sexuality. The flat is beautifully decorated, with cats lying around everywhere, who come up to nuzzle and be stroked, or just lie in the sun. She has bought a packet of biscuits specially for my visit and it is there throughout our talk tempting and accusing her. She mentions that she'd like me to eat some or she will eat them all later, and I feel that the biscuits begin to take on a life and symbolism of their own. Where I see a packet of fancy chocolate biscuits, Annie sees struggle, temptation and wickedness.

Caroline

Seventy-three. She is stalwart of the Women's Institute. Real coffee is served in elegant cups. An affectionate dog is curled on the back of the sofa and wheezes periodically.

I stopped having periods very suddenly when my husband left me. It was a sort of shock reaction and they never started again. I was forty-four. I certainly went through the hot flushes. I had them about twelve years, they just seemed to go on indefinitely. I had them in the day time and they went on for ages. I just put up with them. I went to the doctor but nothing very helpful was ever suggested. There wasn't any HRT then. That was the worst feature as far as I was concerned. They were an awful nuisance.

You can feel it coming up, you can feel a terrific flush rising, you feel you might burst, and then it suddenly subsides again. It can be very embarrassing when you're out with other people you don't know very well. You go red, it is a literal flush, you know it's coming and you know there is nothing you can do about it, you have to bear it. And you look at everybody in the room and you think can everyone see? It's an unpleasant feeling. I never had it at night though.

As for mood swings, it is very difficult to tell what was the menopause and what was my situation. When I went through menopause you didn't think about it, it wasn't talked about so much, you just didn't consider what was happening to you.

I never talked to my mother about it, I've not the faintest idea what her menopause was like, she would never have talked about it.

Caroline meets me at the station on a warm, sunny day. We drive through country lanes to reach her house, overlooking a typical English park. People are walking their dogs, children are chasing each other – a picture book cameo of English life. I half expect Miss Marple to come walking past the window. But this is modern Britain after all, Caroline's husband is making bread in the kitchen, classical music is coming from the radio. As we talk, it becomes clear that this very conventional, intelligent, educated woman has not, in fact, lived the life she might have expected. Instead it has been full of pain and drama. She seems still slightly puzzled by the turn her life has taken.

Florrie

Eighty-four. She is recovering from a serious road accident, but she is nevertheless full of good humour. Her warm Lancastrian voice welcomes me, tea is made by an invisible acolyte, who has also made the traditional ham sandwiches which we munch as we talk. Homemade scones are lying invitingly on a plate for later.

I stopped having a period and that was it, round about fifty. I didn't have any sort of trouble. The first girl I had when I was forty-one and the next one at forty-four. I didn't know anything about menopause, I'd heard people say about bad reactions and was a bit worried but nothing happened. I didn't have any particular expectations, I was a busy person with young children of course.

I was nearly seventeen before I had a period, and of course mother was very worried about that so she took me to the doctor. I had no idea what we were going up there for because I was feeling quite well! I don't know what he told her but it must have been a great relief for her. I think she thought I had found out some way to have sex and not get pregnant, which she wished she knew probably! So she took me off to the doctors to find out. But we couldn't talk about it directly. I didn't know anything about sex, I've only thought about it in the years since. They were worried about the neighbours, in case you got into trouble – that was the big worry!

The terraced house is on a busy road in a town that has changed enormously in the last fifty years. Florrie was born and bred here and talks about all the changes to the town she loves. She's in pain from being knocked down by a car outside her house and she struggles to find a comfortable position on the sofa. The ham sandwiches piled high on the plate remind me of childhood; perfectly cut bread, a thin layer of butter spread on them and good chunks of ham squashed between the layers. Florrie believes in doing things properly, we have serviettes and knives and plates and the teapot seems to hold endless quantities of strong, northern tea. There is a deep sense of peace in the house.

Dot

Seventy. She is tall, elegant and relaxed, clearly a person at ease with herself. It's a hot day and cold spread lunch is already set out on little dishes when I arrive mid-morning.

I went through a sort of rebirth at menopause. Looking back now it was a very tough time, but I was also looking after myself, taking up things that I knew were right for me, like going to yoga. Then, by accident, I fell into the hands of a healer when I hurt my back and then I got involved in healing and that took me into counselling and then I really had to come to terms with myself. I learnt the whole bit about myself and what had made me come to this state of almost breakdown and began to surface. That's thirteen years ago.

I went through menopause at fifty-seven. It was pretty tough, I don't know why, I seemed to imagine it would be. I retired so that I wouldn't have it during my working life. The doctors said this is breaking all the rules at fifty-seven. I felt I was going to have some form of breakdown, so I might as well have it in comfort, rather than still be working.

I knew retirement would be hard because I was so much in demand at work and then the physical symptoms of menopause were also horrific, the usual ones, the sweats. I went into another bedroom and I said, 'I'm not coming back until I'm capable of coping with this'.

I had been on tranquillisers a long time. I had been coming off them almost all my life. I had given up smoking a long time earlier and then I started trying to give up the drugs, thinking I am going to be drug free. So I was really fighting three battles at the same time. I knew I had to get through it. I was on Librium for yonks, since they were invented, and I was never told they were addictive. And sleeping tablets, heavily drugged to keep me going. It wasn't depression, it was all for anxiety. I had several ulcers. I had lots to be anxious about, I had become an anxiety type by then.

Anyone looking at me would have said this was a hugely successful person, but I know that I wore a very good mask and I look for the mask on everybody now because I think we all wear them. I don't want to be known as that person any more, it was a very good act and I was very capable at doing it. I don't think I ever wilfully played a part, I gave my job my whole heart and being. I was able to do that in compensation for the loving that I wasn't able to give in other ways. I have no regrets. I'm more me now.

Life has just become happier and happier for me as far as years are concerned. I've come into being a person for the first time in all my seventy years.

Dot confused me. Here was this elegant, capable woman, the sort of person who could organise a sit-down meal for five hundred, all with different dietary needs and not bat an eyelid. Someone you would instinctively trust, a natural leader, one of the competent organisers in life. She could make a date with you in Ulan Bator in three months time at ten past three, under the clock in the main square, and you know she would be there. And here she was telling me it had all been built on sand, that her inner life was a complete mess, in terrible turmoil and that she had only begun to come out of it when she deliberately retired early. She had realised that she must do battle with her demons, and in her quiet, competent way, had set herself up to do just that.

Maud

Seventy-eight. She is a bright, sparky, well-dressed woman. She thinks carefully before answering my questions and has a wicked sense of humour.

I was fifty-two when I went through menopause. It wasn't terrible at all, I'm a great believer in the fact that you can dismiss a lot of ailments if you don't take too much notice of them. At the moment I'm having this awful back trouble and I've had endless accidents, maybe I'm being taught that that is not so! I tried to disregard my menopause and I didn't suffer from any of the hot flushes or any of those things. I had quite a bit of flooding just before the end, and after that it just cleared up. I was highly delighted.

My mother never talked about things like that, certainly not! I had various friends who'd been going through it. I'm always terribly sorry for people who have a hard time. My daughter, she's now fifty-four and she has been going through it now for a while and she's had a bad time. I think I was very lucky. Some of it is psychological. I was just looking forward to the end of it all, and I was rather annoyed when I got these floodings – I didn't think that was fair at all! I was looking forward to the end of periods, partly because I never enjoyed any part of them, messy business, and also I think it was because I was free not to worry about sex.

I can't believe this bright, attractive woman is nearly eighty. She's smartly dressed; beautifully cut trousers, a nice blouse and silk scarf flowing round her shoulders. She's been to the hairdresser and her make-up is discreet and tasteful. When I ask her some questions, one of her eyebrows shoots up humorously while she thinks of the answer. She's clearly had and given a lot of enjoyment in her life, it shines out of her. If you suggested taking the night train to Istanbul, the gleam in her eye makes you think she might just take you up on it. She leans forward in her chair when she answers, keen that I should understand her exact meaning.

Mary

Forty-seven. A slim blonde comes to the door and I assume it is the daughter of the person I've come to see. I'm shocked to discover she is only a few years older than me. She looks tired, with the tiredness that long illness brings, but she has a warm smile.

I was forty-five. I said to my husband that if HRT had not been available, they would have had to have taken me away. I really believe that. When I hear that women went mad in the past through menopause, I understand exactly why. They weren't actually going mad, it was just everything crowding in and you're trying to struggle through all this alone at home. I couldn't have gone to work to save my life.

I had a back operation which caused a thrombosis. Then I had a hysterectomy because I had a fibroid. Because of the thrombosis, when I had the hysterectomy, they couldn't put me on HRT and because of that basically I went through twenty months of menopause symptoms. It was like having an accelerated menopause. My doctor said that instead of going into it gently, I just hurtled in, which is exactly how it felt. They couldn't help me in any way.

There were panic attacks, loss of memory, exhaustion and fatigue, vaginal dryness, mouth ulcers virtually every other week. Because I was so low, my body couldn't fight anything and it ended last year with me having pneumonia. Hot flushes in bed, that was very bad, it was worse at night than it was in the day time.

I was very depressed and you can't bring yourself out of it. You're tired, so therefore you can't do the things you want to do, that you've always done. It's like living in someone else's body, that was how I described it to the gynaecologist.

Just generally lack of interest, getting up and wanting to do something and then suddenly it all goes. Memory loss is terrible, that is one of the worst things. You go into a shop or into the supermarket and you're fine, then suddenly you find yourself just standing there and it's like someone is draining it all out of your head. You just stand there thinking 'What am I doing here? What did I come in here for?'

I had terrible panic attacks, mostly when I was out. In your own home, you can wander round the house, until your brain comes back into gear, but when you're in a shop, if you just stand stock still in the middle of a supermarket and start gazing at people, they just don't understand at all, people just stare at you. I found if I'd got something to look at I was OK. So I would take a list, sometimes I would just pick something up, anything, and walk out. Usually I would have to come home or walk for a while before I could start to think what I actually wanted, before I could start to calm down.

I got a lot of help from the gynaecologist. The doctor wasn't very good, she didn't want me to go on HRT. The gynaecologist didn't see why I shouldn't, so I was caught in between the both of them. She thought it was dangerous, he knew it was dangerous but he monitored me and I trusted him. He was just so good and reassuring, the one person I would say, outside of my family, that I could really talk to.

No one told me it would be this bad. I read all the books, I joined the Amarant trust. I was convinced it was menopause, even when I was going through it. I thought this must be what it is. But nothing prepares you for how you're going to feel, nothing at all. The gynaecologist said things will pass and it will get better.

When you're going through it, you feel totally alone because you're thinking, 'what about all these other people who are suffering?' They either won't own up to the fact that they are old enough for the menopause, or they just don't want to talk. I can't understand it, where are they all, it can't be just me?

I was a changed person. In a way I think my husband quite liked it because I used to sit down and was no longer this person zooming about the place, getting something done. But obviously he didn't like to see me upset. Since I've got myself back to near what I was before, he's getting a bit desperate because I'm all over the place decorating and doing all those sorts of things again.

I could explain to him how bad I was feeling and to my mother – she was a big help. I'd got them both, my mum and my husband, but nobody else. They are the people who are going to believe you. When you start to talk to someone, you can see a look come on their face and they are either going to listen to you or they aren't. And the majority of people aren't. So you stop talking, you stop saying anything. My mother hadn't had a difficult menopause, but she could see what I was suffering and she was with me quite a lot. We'd go out shopping and she could see that I was exhausted, more tired than I have ever been in my life, she just knew that things were bad.

It's HRT that's helped. A positive attitude which I've tried to have all along hasn't worked. They put me on HRT after three months, but very low dosages. I had a patch which took away the night sweats and the hot flushes, but it didn't help with anything else much. Now I'm on a fairly high dose. When I first went on the higher dose, it was just this positive feeling, I felt that everything was going to be fine. So I went raving mad doing everything then realised that my body will only take so much because it is not only the menopause but all the other health factors I'm getting over and the emotional stuff too of course.

HRT really, really helped. It can't be anything else because it has been a gradual feeling. I've noticed how much more I can do now, but I am starting to realise what my capabilities and limitations are. As for coping emotionally with it, what I did was to deny it all. That was probably part of the trouble. I knew someone who was diagnosed with cancer about the same time I damaged my back, and I just kept thinking 'You're better off than she is, you're better off than everybody else, pull yourself together. You're all right, you've got your family and you are going to get better.' But there were many days, when even though I said that to myself, I still thought I can't handle this. And then somebody said to me that I was trivialising my illness too much. She said it was fine to count my blessings, but I was ill and had been very ill. So I felt I was caught in the middle all the time.

Nobody suggested counselling. I did think about it, but then I thought, what can they tell me that I don't know already? It wasn't a mystery, I knew exactly what it was and what was going to happen. I was depressed about feeling old. I feel and look a lot better now, because the exhaustion has gone and now I am bothering with myself. There were times when I would do myself up and someone would say, 'Are you all right? You look really tired', and it would just finish it. All that bother and they can tell that I'm not well! It all shows in your face, and of course I lost weight. The depression is bad and you do age because of the memory loss. I literally felt like I was doddering about.

I've always been so organised, but it got to the stage where I'd just throw things together. One day I made a jelly and chocolate flavour blancmange and I just messed both of them up, something I've been making for years! My son came in as I happened to make it. I slopped this blancmange into the dish, all it was was this blob, and I was standing thinking what have I done? He said, 'You've not put enough milk in that'. As we put the spoon in, it leapt out of the dish and bounced across the room! I can laugh about it now, but then I just couldn't believe it at all. Sometimes I just wanted to sit down and cry because I was quite desperate, but if I had it would have made him realise just how bad I was and I didn't want my son to know that, although I think he guessed, he's very sensitive.

I was a young woman still. You just have to take it day to day. You know what you are capable of, so you try and push yourself just that little bit more. I really just thought that everything was finished, I couldn't see a future. It's just in the past month or so really that I can actually look ahead and think, well I have got a future and there are things I can do. I am feeling better and better all the time, but it's been three years of hell.

Mary's terrible menopause shocked me. Her experience of illness and depression seemed too much for one human being to bear. As her story emerges in the book, it's clear that her menopause is only the latest in a long line of tragedy and bad luck. She is the person who first makes me wonder whether difficulties in life somehow come up again during menopause. This is not to attach any blame, simply that maybe a person stores up terrible life experiences which haven't been completely sorted out. Then they emerge as particularly strong physical and mental symptoms at menopause, forcing the woman to stop and look at her life. Mary's home has the spotless, freshly decorated look of the compulsive homemaker; everything in its place, looking sparkling and neat.

Sally

Fifty-two. She is an artist, and she's just had a show in her house. We sit in her kitchen. She's one of those people that seem so familiar, you feel you have known them forever.

All my life, I had been different weights and in different moods and situations, but I had always felt like me. But suddenly I was a different me. I suppose it started when I was forty-six, with stiffness and a general feeling of 'dis-ease'. I had a bad menopause but there were mitigating circumstances; difficulty with my job, a lot of changes with the children, problems with their health and my son's mental health made it hard for me to see the wood for the trees.

Physically, having had relatively painful but regular heavy periods all my adult life, I began to get dysfunctional bleeding. It was a bit of a magical mystery tour, being offered hysterectomy, laser treatment and all that. A doctor friend of mine said it was like a motorbike whose engine had stopped and you would give it a kick start and it would splutter into life, which would cause these very heavy bleeds, and very irregular with it. In fact I was wearing padded pads eventually and taking a towel with me to sit on other people's sofas. It probably went on like that for about four years. Then they began to peter out, and then after six months I'd get a deluge. And although I'd always suffered from PMT, before my periods, I would now have absolute blackness and be dangerous with a bottle of wine – two glasses of wine and I would be away, ready for a fight!

I didn't really realise that I was menopausal because I didn't get the classic hot flushes – I thought this was a menstruation/hormonal problem. I had no picture of my mother's menopause as she had a hysterectomy at thirty-five, so I didn't recognise it immediately. I wasn't enraged at menopause, but I was certainly enraged about being older; fifty was a watershed. There was a rage about my feelings and a fear of being whacky. I certainly wasn't worried about no longer being fertile. But it was the idea of revolution, literally in the change, the panic that seemed to come at fifty.

When the panic came, it would wash over me. Other things happened as well, like I lost a lot of teeth. Then once you're through that, you're not panicking about the state of fifty, you're panicking about sixty, seventy, eighty and then the curtain, it was a panic about death.

Also, I had my children young, but because of circumstances like being a single parent, they had not left; they were still hanging around. I felt rage that I was still having to carry their complexities and unhappiness which I realise now can happen at any point in life. Because I had looked after them with no support, it had been a long and troubled journey and I think I felt, 'Christ, I'm fifty and my life has been tied up with them and their needs and there has been no room for myself as a woman. And here I am no longer fertile but still having to be a mum.'

'If it's not a dependency, it doesn't matter so much, it's part of life. It's when you feel they are hanging on to your skirt and pulling you down like lead weights that it is difficult. During that period with children, nurturing, being two parents, there is no space in that for exploration of your sexuality.

I tried HRT because I thought it would help me to regulate my periods and also with this dysfunctional, all-over feeling I had. I remember the day I started taking it, I thought I was going to grow a beard and my voice was going to drop! I did it quite ceremoniously. Also I had incredible vagueness and it was supposed to temper that. But it was difficult to tell if it really helped, as that year my daughter was in a terrible car crash, so how could I see if it made things better, when things in my life were visibly worse?

I was taking a cyclical pill and I took them the wrong way round by accident because of my vagueness. When I rang up my GP, he suggested stopping for a while, to be back to normal and I thought, 'What is normal? I wasn't normal before and I don't feel normal now!' At that point I'd read a lot about it and I decided that I would try and get through in other ways and I put myself on a massive vitamin programme, quite a structured regime, and since then I have not felt inclined to take it.

There are things about HRT I don't like, this thing of being limber and not having dried-up vaginas, all that sounds to me like men trying to keep women looking as though they are fertile. People say your skin looks good, your hair looks good on HRT, but no one is giving a man HRT to stop him getting wrinkles! So I almost want to be a wizened sexy woman!

Has menopause changed the way I feel about myself? I feel better, there's a relief there. I've had more sex since menopause and I've related to men more strongly, but they have been young men.

Menopause is more than aging; it's a change and moving off. I felt out of kilter completely, I felt very low, I was stiff, it was a horrible time. I've come through it now, finally, at fifty-two. I'm not cyclical any more, so that puts you on almost the same level as a man. It's not that I feel more manly, I feel like a warrior now, more powerful.

Sally was the one person who had no problems answering my questions, indeed trying to get a question in edgeways took all my interviewing skills! Her conversation is an intelligent stream of consciousness, with ideas sparking off other thoughts and memories. She had clearly thought deeply about her life situation and the sexual politics of menopause. She's someone who has finally taken control of her life and who does not trust the experts to tell her what to do. She's also the type of person who clips endless articles from newspapers and magazines, with an informal filing system in her head. Any general topic of conversation will produce a rummage through a sheaf of papers, with a triumphant grin when the right piece is found. She rang me the next day to continue the conversation; our talk had sparked off a lot of thoughts in her.

Jenny

Fifty-four. She is divorced with three children. She is smartly dressed in a warm peach jumper and slacks. She curls her legs up under her on the sofa, at ease with herself. We drink coffee and munch wholewheat biscuits.

It's difficult to say when I started menopause because I was taking HRT. I started taking HRT when I was about forty-eight and then I stopped it for a while just to see what was happening. It was quite straightforward; I used to get a bit irritable at times, but no other real problems. I took HRT for the hot flushes and also because both my mother and my aunt had osteoporosis. Menopause took about three years – not long.

Not being fertile any more has never been an issue that I've confronted at all; it has never bothered me. A lot of people do, I know, feel quite emotional about it.

I'm a believer in HRT, very much so, I feel so very much better when I am on it. I'm less tired, I just feel brighter altogether. I've been on my own for four years now. When I came off it I did get quite low and depressed but that was my state of mind in any case, so it's difficult to tell how I would have felt otherwise. But I've certainly found it easier to cope with the problems I've had over the years, when I've been on HRT. I take it for three weeks and then one week off and at one stage during the week off I used to get very low, but it doesn't seem so bad now.

Menopause wasn't ever something that I dwelt on because I have always been busy and worked in my life. Some women dread it, I know, but it was never a big issue with me – ever. I didn't really notice it at all.

Last year I did go through quite a patch of having to confront the fact that I was getting older – in my mid-fifties – and I didn't like that much at all. I'm a different person now. I'm more confident and much, much calmer. It is nice not to get PMT every month because I really did get it dreadfully badly for three weeks every month! It's wonderful not to have all these terrible ups and downs as I'm fairly placid and laid back really.

I've probably made a lot more friends since menopause than I have made all my life. I don't know whether it's because I'm on my own, because when you are a couple you function as a couple. I've had to make new friends – no way was I going to sit down and be a nothing. I've loosened up a bit too, it's strange. My life is richer now in lots of ways, although there is a big gap since my divorce.

My mother always put me down – nobody will ever want to listen to you, you are no good – and you do believe it, so you don't make friends. You back off people all the time if you've always been told that you're useless . . . I can remember my mother saying nobody will ever love you. It's such a destructive thing to say to a child, and you carry that all your life. But now I have got rid of it. It was a huge effort and took a lot of determination. Here I was getting on for fifty and I jolly well wasn't going to ruin the rest of my life with it.

My marriage broke up during menopause. I was very angry and I do wonder sometimes, how much of the anger at my husband was due to the menopause. It's hard to tell when you're going through difficulties in your marriage in any case. But I'm not angry now, so I do wonder. I couldn't keep my mouth shut! I was so angry and het up that I just had to say it. Just like having PMT – you get so screwed up, you have got to come out with it regardless.

Probably I was angry at my childhood that wasn't particularly easy either. I was very angry with my mother. Also, I suppose subsconsciously I was angry that my husband had an affair, I was furious about that. So the two together just seemed to be coming out at menopause. It's a good question – why I had I lived with those emotions all those years?

It wasn't an anger that was directed at the outside world, no one outside my home would have known at all. Something about the menopause allowed me to deal with those feelings. Also my mother was getting older – she was eighty-eight when she died – and as she got older you could see the nastiness in her, which I lived through as child, coming out again. I thought, 'I've got to confront this before she dies, it's no good doing it when they are gone'.

My husband probably reacted because I was so angry and so verbal, perhaps this is what drove him away to someone else. It was stuff that had been bottled up for years, anger that I had had against my mother all my life, I directed at him as I couldn't do it to her. He couldn't understand what was going on at all. I felt guilty about the anger but I just couldn't help it, I really couldn't. I'd come out with ridiculous things like the way he boiled the eggs! I'd come down and if the water wasn't boiling I used to really carry on, it was awful! I wouldn't behave like that now, it was a very specific stage, I had a change of personality, carrying on about boiled eggs!

Menopause definitely heightened all those emotions, so everything I felt, I felt more strongly. The me of five years before wouldn't have said anything at all about the eggs. I just exploded about everything, when I think about it now it is quite horrendous. I hated the changes in me, absolutely hated them, but I just couldn't seem to stop myself.

I knew that I had to resolve the difficulties with my mother before I could get on with my life again, so I did have a lot of counselling and that also changed how I perceived myself. My mother died two years ago. I see menopause as a time of now or never, it was quite a transition. It wasn't easy feeling like I did, with a young child, because I had my youngest at forty-two so she was only about eight or nine then.

It gets a bit boring sleeping with the same person for twenty years! It can do. He was a very introspective, quiet sort of person and I'm not basically. My expectations did change over the years, the passion did die down, particularly on his part, and I thought 'Blow me, I don't want this to just trickle down into nothing after twenty years. I've still got a long time to live!'

No, I didn't accept it at all and that was some of the problem, it wasn't easy to deal with. He was made redundant and totally lost interest in sex. I was quite understanding, I realised men do get impotent when they go through problems, but even before that he was beginning to lose interest and just jog along in his own sweet way. I've been on my own for four years now.

Jenny lives in a quiet cul-de-sac outside Durham. The house feels lived in and cheerful with a small, sunny garden out back. It's difficult to reconcile the woman sitting here in front of me, in her fashionable clothes and enthusiastic conversation, with her past. But when she talks about her mother, it's clearly still a painful subject. Her teenage daughter arrives home from school at the end of our conversation and the talk turns to Neighbours *and who is doing what to whom. Then the conversation turns to that evening and the disco and which pair of jeans are exactly right to wear. Jenny takes her daughter's anguish (at precisely who else will be there and what they will be wearing) seriously. It's delightful to see the warm, positive relationship she has with her daughter.*

Jenny is typical of many women – menopause was a time when she had to reassess her life and get help to cope with damage done to her earlier in life. The confusion in her life seemed to come from several sources; problems with her mother, her husband's affair, a young child and suffering so badly at menopause as she had with PMT over the years. It's difficult to believe that this calm woman could once have been the harpy that she describes with some humour. Jenny has clearly come through the tunnel of menopause into a different, more positive life.

Mavis

Seventy-three. The flat, on the fifth floor of a council block, is cheerful and bright. Fashionably dressed with stylish hair, Mavis looks fifteen years younger than her age.

It didn't change the way I felt about myself, I wouldn't allow it to. It's one of those things, part of your life, part of growing up. You've got to keep yourself attractive.

My menopause was fairly easy, no problem at all. I didn't have any bad floodings, I missed a couple of periods and I was a bit panicky, because in those days one did panic. I didn't have any traumatic experience at all except that I lost all my hair, which was a tremendous shock. That lasted fourteen months and they said it was a hormone deficiency and my hair would never come back again, but it did without any problem at all.

I suppose menopause took about five or six years but I'm sure that in those days we didn't make a fuss about it. There didn't seem time to think, 'Oh God I've got a period', or a headache, or something else. That's what I feel today, when I talk to some of the young people my daughter's age. They've got stacks of little pills, they take them for one reason or another and everything is going to be better; they think it's going to keep them young. Both my grandmother and my mother used the philosophy, if you got up in the morning and didn't feel well, you would go to school and you would be all right. I have been like that all my life and I think that too many people today make excuses.

At one stage, when I was having dripping periods for weeks, it got on my nerves and I was very glad when it was all over, because it does go on a bit. But maybe I was lucky because I never felt ill at all. HRT wasn't available, but I don't think I would have taken it, but who knows, times have changed over the last ten years.

I didn't feel it was a big stage in my life. You knew it was going to happen, you knew everything was going to change, but there was never any big drama about it, never. I always kept up my appearance, I always have. It's an absolute stupidity when I see some women who directly they get to the menopause they become old ladies, they really do.

It's all in the mind, at least my mother used to tell me that. She was always very open about what happened. My mother had a child during menopause. She didn't realise she was pregnant, she thought it was the change of life and she went to the doctor who said she was four months' pregnant. At that time I realised that I was expecting my daughter too!

I don't think any of us knew what to expect. A lot of people made a big fuss about it, moaning about not being able to have any more children and that sort of thing. From my point of view, I never wanted any more children so that was fine. I was glad to get it all over and done with. From the sexual point of view, menopause was great because I didn't have to worry, at least you knew you couldn't be pregnant, you could go away any time that you wanted to. It made things better.

Mavis had bought some little cakes for tea and tucked into them with the confidence of someone at ease with themselves. We had proper cups and saucers, she believes in style and doing things properly. She, of all the women I spoke to, confounds my prejudice about age. She's up to date with current affairs, keen and bright, and refuses to be categorised as an elderly woman. When I leave, she suggests we go out for a pizza sometime and I'm flattered that she feels I'm young enough!

Madeleine

Seventy-three. A warm, smiling face greets me at the door of a comfortable house a few miles outside Manchester. Clearly she is a person happy in her skin. Her husband chats easily with me while she makes coffee.

I probably went through menopause in my late forties. I had a D and C because I had such terribly heavy periods and then when I was about forty-five, forty-six, they put me on HRT to try and control this, but I felt so groggy that I gave it up. I did get hot sweats for years and years – hot all over. It's quite funny really, you've been in company and say, 'Gosh, it's hot in here' and they say, 'Well no it isn't really!' I've always had quite heavy periods, but they got worse and worse as I got older.

I didn't particularly have mood swings, not that I was aware of, but Christopher says there was that slight irritability at some times; it maybe made me a little bit short-tempered but it didn't affect anybody really.

HRT made me dizzy. I wasn't well at all at the time and the doctor said he could give me another pill to stop the dizziness. I was not having all that, but I've gone back to HRT just a month or so ago – people know what they are doing now. I've met a few women who are on it and they have a sparkle and of course it stops your bones dissolving. They can judge the dosages better now.

I had a cousin who was almost in a mental home at that time because of her menopause and there were others who had horrendous times, so I knew there was a big range of different experiences. But I had nothing really upsetting, maybe a bit tearful more often than I would be normally, but thinking back on it, it was nothing to comment about really.

It seems there is a range, from not even noticing that it had stopped to this poor woman who was really mental. I presume it was all hormones whizzing around and we are all different. Also this person didn't have any children – not that she thought very deeply about it, but maybe behind that was a thought, 'Well I never will now'.

Of course, by the end of menopause, my children had grown up, because I was married at twenty and my son was born at twenty-one. If I'd had littles ones I might have felt differently about it, but to me I'd lived an awful long while being a mother.

Madeleine has a quality of stillness and peace around her. The house is in a smart area, with beautiful trees overhanging the garden. The sitting room is comfortable, with lots of easy chairs – it has that lived-in look about it that makes you want to stay and have another cup of coffee. She refers to herself as having been pretty, but she is still very beautiful, with the sort of looks that grow on you even more the longer you're with her. But it's the quality of her presence that is striking; she radiates happiness and an inner calm.

Alice

Sixty. We meet in her office and she comes bustling in, organising coffee and the chairs. She is very smartly dressed. She is also a bit nervous when we start.

I had an early menopause in my late forties but I didn't recognise it as that. I had a lot of depressions and sweating – I've been on anti-depressants often with all the problems I've had. It was my forward-thinking GP who put me on HRT and that helped, but I started bleeding after a few years and I could see myself using my bus pass to go and get my Tampax, which I really didn't relish! So I came off HRT and I've been on and off it since. I'm using primrose oil now and I'm fine.

I wasn't angry, it buoyed me up tremendously because I was going to be given a pill that might help me, which it did of course. I had no sense of loss though. There's a lot of self-esteem wrapped up in this because I was very active, I was a chairman of magistrates, which I still am, and I'm still active in Relate, even though I had a rough old rotten marriage myself.

I'd never talked about menopause to anyone, hadn't even thought about it. The only reason to think about menopause is if you've got a sexually active life – whoopee you don't have to bother with contraception anymore. I'd had so many problems and worries that I didn't think about it.

Alice is one of life's organisers. Even the way she comes into the room says here is a person who can and will take charge. We meet at her office and it's only subsequently that I understand why. Her public and private life are completely separate. She's a heavy smoker, working in a non-smoking environment, and is proud of the fact that she can go all day without a cigarette. She smokes on the way in and on the way home and doesn't even sneak out for one in the park opposite, like the rest of the staff – typical of her strong-willed determination.

Clare

Fifty-six. She is a slim, fashionably dressed woman who perches nervously on her chair and seems a bit wary at first.

I went through menopause at forty-nine, fifty. It wasn't too traumatic; mood swings, the usual flushes and what have you. About five years ago I went onto HRT, which I think has helped a lot, and although it has its drawbacks, basically the menopausal symptoms went. I'm on a much more even keel.

I had wild mood swings; in a matter of an hour you could be right up and then it was over, or else terribly low. It wasn't really unusual for me, but it did accentuate how I felt normally. It was hard for me, but even worse for my husband. At least I knew, let me storm around or whatever, or be terribly low and depressed and it will pass.

It was a rite of passage, one that you wouldn't really desire to have because it made it more difficult for my husband. And I like to feel even and calm and serene and able to cope all the time, without flying off the handle over something I normally would not have done. I didn't see it as an end of life – emotionally it didn't upset me too much, the thought that my childbearing years were over.

Clare appears younger than her age and very nervous. She spends the first twenty minutes squirming on her chair and sipping at her coffee. As she becomes more relaxed, she smiles more. She's obviously been working herself up for our interview, thinking over her life and the various problems she has had, and I wonder why she agreed to it. Throughout our time together, I'm struck by her honesty in reply to my questions, however painful they are at times, as she hesitates for a moment and then plunges in with her reply. Her husband comes into the conversation very early. She's obviously very much in love with him and thinks of herself all the time in relation to him. He is her point of reference.

Brenda

Fifty-four. She is a cheerful, bundle of energy. She's clearly very happy with her life, and she smiles and bubbles with good humour as we talk.

I did not want to go through the change. It symbolises pain and discomfort, dowdiness, falling into a pattern. I see that in all the friends that are my age; it seems to take their sparkle away. I think that's basically it, it just takes their sparkle away, gives them an excuse not to do things any more. An acceptance that they're in that menopausal state and that gives them the freedom to be as they are expected to be.

It just felt there was nothing about it that was going to be good; you got osteoporosis, you had hot flushes, your skin was going to dry up, your vagina was going to dry up. I went to the opticians and my bloody eyes were drying up! [*She laughs.*] I felt it was totally negative, I was putting on weight, not that I had a big bust, just everything seemed to be dropping.

I started menopause when I was about fifty. Before that I had the hot flushes, but I wouldn't accept it, no way! Everybody else had hot flushes, I just was hot! [*She laughs again.*] Luckily it happened mostly at night and I didn't tell anybody or recognise it; that went on for two or three years.

A friend of mine had gone through the change quite early in life – I'd seen her go through it – and she'd had to have tablets for her nerves. I was determined I was not going to go any tablets. I was going to be totally different from everyone else. I suppose if I'm honest, I don't like tablets – I wouldn't go on the pill, for example. I was determined that I wasn't going to be the norm.

I accepted the fact after a while that perhaps these were hot flushes and the fact that I was getting up three or four times a night absolutely soaking wet. I thought, 'Well, perhaps I'm going in for the change here!' I went to the doctor, but I didn't say I was having hot flushes. I told her I was getting hot at night, so she said that's hot flushes. She just said go on HRT. I felt there must be another way I could handle it, so I asked if I could I go to a specialist and talk it through, because I didn't like the fact of someone just giving you tablets. I asked her if she shouldn't do blood tests, talk to me. Plus the fact that my mum has had breast cancer.

She gave me a couple of books – obviously I was taking up too much of her time – and said come back. So I took the books away and thought, 'I'm not happy with this', so I then went through a phase when I said, 'This is not happening'.

The hot sweats carried on, and I still get them now. Then I was getting a little bit edgy. I don't know if it was because I'd read this book – you might get edgy, you might get this – so I thought, 'Hang on I'm conforming to the norm', so I really fought against all these symptoms.

I was angry at having to go through these things at a time of life when I should be enjoying myself. I thought it was too early, I think sixtyish would have been better. Growing old and still feeling young, this was the crux of it, there's so much I wanted to do and I just felt that if I took one inkling that that was the change, it would slow me down and I was determined that no way was anything like this going to slow me down. But it is the change!

It hasn't slowed me down. I have a lot of friends of similar ages and we meet regularly every month. We've developed since we were young wives – six to eight of us meet. We've been doing that for the last twenty-five years, all the children growing up, should we tell them about the pill, etc. There's been a different cross section of us and I've seen them age quite rapidly. Most of the women are on HRT. I didn't feel that it made them any brighter or any better. They seemed to accept the fact that they had to go through all of this and they thought I was a bit stupid – the pill's there so why don't you take it, it's a good opportunity. I suppose I've dealt with it in the best way for me.

I don't think my mother had too bad a menopause. She was quite late, but she just went through it. I've got a negative image of menopause, mainly because of the people I've seen; this feeling that at fifty-four you've got to expect it, you're menopausal. The way they dress is different, more staid, they sit back to an older image. A lot of them suddenly go on to part-time work, they were holding down full-time jobs and they felt it was time to ease back. Even how they looked, they were quite happy to go grey, not to bother quite so much. It didn't bother *them* doing it, I think it bothered *me* their doing it.

My concern is still osteoporosis if I don't take HRT. But I love not having periods; they're a bore, messy. I'd feel so unclean and the dragging pain, so that's really been good. Total liberation, and that's given me a freedom that's good.

Brenda was a strange mixture. She greeted me rather shyly and I thought it was going to be difficult to get her to speak frankly. But she turned out to be the person who talked most openly about her life and her sexuality. She also had me roaring with laughter at some of her descriptions. She describes a happy, conventional, suburban life with great good humour. I think she rather likes the idea that she is not as ordinary as she seems on the outside; there's a gleam in her eye that suggests mischief!

Judith

Sixty-two. She lives in a pretty village in the country. She is welcoming and hospitable.

I had a hysterectomy in 1979. I don't think it changed my sex life at all, if anything it enhanced it, probably through not worrying about getting pregnant. Also there was the fact that my hormones were more stable and I was less emotional. I seemed to enjoy it more and perhaps I was more relaxed about it in every way.

As you get older, I don't think sex changes a great deal. You gain expertise, obviously, and you are more relaxed and confident in being able to please your partner and you get more out of it yourself.

Judith is typical of many women of her generation; shy and reserved on the outside, with a rich inner life. She took some persuading that her opinions mattered or were of interest, but then showed that she had thought carefully about many of the issues under discussion. As the eldest of several children, she felt responsible for her elderly mother who was beginning to depend on her more and more to take decisions on her behalf. She'd recently retired and been asked back part time, which made her feel needed and valued. She lives in a picture postcard English village in a house decorated with care.

Katherine

Fifty-three. She is dressed in a shortish check skirt and pale green cashmere jumper with a coral necklace. Appearance is important to her. She thinks carefully before she speaks at her office, where she is the boss.

My husband is six years older than I am, but feels that he's a lot older than that. He's always been concerned about the way I look, so, almost to a point of selfishness, he wants me to be like a trophy as it were. I wondered if he was going to worry about menopause, but he didn't seem to worry about it at all and was very supportive, in fact encouraged me to find out about my hormone levels and HRT, obviously because he'd like me to go on looking young for a bit longer.

I feel a lot more self-secure; I feel if I don't want to do that, then why the hell should I, and whether it's menopause, or simply that I've been working more since the kids grew up and moved away, I don't know. I'm more self-sufficient.

A lot of things changed in my sexuality but I don't know if it was incidental, or because of work, or just time. I was expecting menopause to affect my sexuality. I don't know whether it's the pills or just the circumstances, but I feel a lot more sexual, or maybe that's part of my new feeling of independence. I was feeling bit towards this way before I started on HRT. It's probably got more to do with my working and being more successful in my job and feeling like I am somebody. But also because of years and years and years of being a housewife, I've had more chance in the last ten years, since I've been working seriously full time, to bounce off younger women and their attitude is fantastic and it's rubbed off on me.

I've actually sat behind a young man on a bus who was wearing a little T shirt with a low neck and the urge to tickle the back of his neck was almost overpowering! And I thought 'Hmm, shall I take you home and give you a seeing to?' But then the worry is that they will look at you and think, 'Yuk you're old'.

When I went to meet Katherine in the lobby of the office building where she works, there were several people waiting. Casting my eyes over them, it was hard to pick out which might be the post-menopausal one. When Katherine came forward with a welcoming smile (I'd described what I would be wearing) I was struck by her appearance and her vivacity. She leant forward on the desk, anxious that I should understand what she meant when she described her life. She was one of the women for whom menopause had been a liberation.

Joan

Fifty-two. She's carefully dressed and a little cautious. She is keen to correct herself if she thinks I haven't understood her.

I would want to say to people that it doesn't need to be as traumatic as sometimes it's portrayed. We don't hear about normal menopause at all. I began menopause at about forty-five. It affected me physically; I felt very tired and had the sweats at night and I found it all very tedious. I feel much better now than I did at forty-five – better physically, more energy. I didn't experience some of the awful mood swings that I know other people have had, or particular tensions either.

I'm single and not in a relationship with anyone so I didn't really resent menopause particularly. I'd come to the conclusion that, even if I were to meet and marry someone, I probably wouldn't have children, so it didn't seem an inordinate thing to happen to me and in a sense I'm quite glad that I've got it over early. When the menopause started, I was actually in a relationship – not a physical one – that meant a lot to me and that was a situation that was more affecting my thoughts on life and where it was going and my age.

I think it's important to separate menopause from the aging process. I suppose because I'm involved in medicine, I'm conscious of the ways in which our body physiologically ages. Chronological aging is quite different and I think the two should be kept separate, although I think each has an influence on the other obviously.

Medically, the menopause is part of the natural life cycle of a woman, not something to be resented – although that's easier said than done – but to be viewed as part of the pattern of living and growth. There are still a few lurking fears that I might get osteoporosis or put on a lot of weight, or some other physical effect, but as time goes on the likelihood of that happening, at least in the near future, is diminishing.

I have to confess to having been rather blinkered about it because I'd heard enough to make me think that it could be upsetting and result in a lot of side-effects and, to be honest with you, I felt that the more I knew about it, the more I had the capacity to become a hypochondriac. So although I knew the basic facts, I didn't indulge in, or purposely read a lot of material about the menopause or what it might do to me. I just carried on with my life.

Joan's house was on a quiet, terraced street. The sitting room was beautifully decorated with her own embroidery, and a lot of thought had clearly gone into her surroundings. We sat at the table in the dining room. She took some time to answer my questions, with long, thoughtful gaps, and I could sense her really trying to respond honestly. But there was a certain guarded caution to her answers initially, the reason becoming clear as we talked and she was keen that I should understand her point of view and principles. There was a certain shyness there too.

Chapter Two

Marriage and long-term relationships

Ignorance isn't bliss, and that is particularly true when it comes to marriage. There is much debate today about how much our children should be taught about sex, whether it should come from parents or school and whether parents should have the right to withdraw their children from sex education. Listening to the women in this book makes it clear that information can only be a good thing and that sex education should be made as compulsory as maths or English. It should, of course, not be taught in a vacuum, after all sex is not some form of mechanical engineering, but in the context of relationships.

So education in conducting relationships, how to maintain them, what to do when they go wrong, is also vital. If we don't expect people to learn how to read or count or drive a car through osmosis, how can we expect children to learn how to form decent and responsible lasting relationships with healthy sexual attitudes if they are not informed and educated?

In this chapter I wanted to find out how marriage and long-term relationships have changed over the different generations. Most of the women I interviewed had been married or in long-term relationships. Several women had been married more than once, and two had married, divorced, remarried, divorced and then got back together with their first husbands! One was married twice and still a virgin when she married for the second time.

I wanted to establish what early expectations of marriage the women had and how those expectations changed. Did they know about sex? Was it possible to maintain a happy sex life over several decades? What happened to the relationship when, for one reason or another, the sex didn't work out?

The youngest woman I interviewed was forty-seven, the oldest eighty-four. Was there any difference in their expectations? The oldest could remember generations before her own; what had their attitudes to sex and marriage been? Did women in their fifties expect more than women in their eighties? Was sexual compatibility essential to a happy marriage and if so, was it chance or something that could be worked at? What happened when a marriage broke down?

In the past, marriage – the ties that bind – was the life most women aspired to and expected. For the older generation, in their seventies and eighties, there was no question of choosing to remain single. Women were bound by the ties of convention; you met a boy you liked and then you married him. And you stayed married. Desperately unhappy marriages had to be withstood – several women were still married to men they should have divorced decades ago. The lack of choice about whom one married was compounded by the almost total ignorance in sexual matters.

Many of the women I spoke to had no information about sex at all when they got married. One woman spoke of a neighbour who had run into the street in her nightdress on her wedding night, screaming that her new husband was trying to attack her; knowing nothing about sex, she thought that it was violence. Many of the new young husbands were as ignorant as their wives, with no notion of a woman's desires or needs. They thought sex was a duty to be performed by the woman, like keeping the house neat and tidy.

Some older women were more fortunate in marrying a man who was more considerate or experienced, or by chance they happened to discover that they were sexually compatible with their husbands.

This generation of women expected nothing from sex, and by and large they got nothing. One woman was married for twelve years to an older man, with whom she had no sexual pleasure, though she describes the marriage as a happy one. When he died, she married again, this time a man with experience who helped her to discover her own sexuality. She has never looked back and now, at over eighty years old, she has a live-in boyfriend in his sixties.

If good sex in marriage is about communication, then many of these marriages were doomed; after all, if the mothers of these women had thought sex too filthy a subject to be mentioned, and the onset of periods a dirty but unavoidable topic, how could these young, shy, virginal wives possibly talk about sex, always assuming they knew they were missing out?

Knowledge was vital, and the one or two women of the older generation who did know about sex got their information from married colleagues at work or from Marie Stopes, the great feminist pioneer whose book *Married Love*, was quoted by several women. It explained that sex should be pleasurable for both partners and gave women a glimmer of hope.

The war years also brought many sexual freedoms, and women admitted to having had affairs while their husbands were away which inevitably gave them a means of comparison. But many remained trapped in loveless marriages. One woman whose family forced her to marry a man she had run away with, but not actually slept with, discovered that she had married a psychopath. She knew her family would believe the respectable front he maintained, so when she did finally run away from him, they would only allow her a separation, not a divorce. The social influence of the family was so strong at that time that she agreed. Looking back on this now, she smiles at my surprise in her submitting to family and social pressure and approves completely of my generation's freedom.

There were several women in their seventies who had had good sexual relationships with their partners. I was intrigued by them – was it just chance or a special relationship that made the difference? In some marriages it seemed that if the husband was experienced and gentle then good lines of communication were established early on. Other women just had a lust for life that carried them through. Many women, now widows, spoke fondly of their husbands as sexual partners.

I was also surprised by the frankness of the older generation. I had been prepared to find them coy about sex or to find it impossible to discuss with a younger woman. But they talked quite freely, though not as graphically, as their younger counterparts. Most of them had never experienced orgasm and they were curious about what it might be like. And some, in their seventies and eighties, still live in hope!

So what education did they give their daughters? Although they found it just as difficult to talk about sex as their mothers had, by the time their daughters were growing up, more information was generally available and women had access to that information through friends and the work place. The great difference in this younger generation was that they went out to work and the world opened up to them. They began to be financially independent so should things go wrong they had the means to leave, whereas the previous generation just had to put up with life. Working meant chatting over lunch, being more open to new ideas in magazines, and being able to compare notes with other women.

Men, too, were more informed, and the women now in their sixties generally seem to have had more pleasure from marriage. Some women were led into disastrous relationships by their sexual desire – one woman described her attraction for colourful wasters with what seemed equal measures of sadness and relish.

Some women in their fifties lived the same lives their mothers had – no communication, sex talk taboo within marriage. But it is this generation of women who have really changed the most in their attitudes to sex and marriage. These women belonged to the first generation to have access to the contraceptive pill, freeing them from the worry of pregnancy and allowing them greater sexual freedom. It's clear that they were much better informed and consequently not trapped by the ignorance of previous generations. They expected sexual pleasure in marriage and were more able to talk about sex with their partners. This led both to closer relationships and happier sex lives, but also to more break-ups as women refused to put up with the unhappy sex lives their mothers had taken as the norm.

The exception is the gay woman in her fifties who still had to deal with hostility, ignorance and prejudice which led to a nervous breakdown. She remembers the difficulty of not being able to come out as being gay, having absolutely no one to talk to, believing that she was the only gay woman in London. She even tried sleeping with men, thinking that she just had to grit her teeth and get on with it; this of course led to an even greater sense of alienation.

One woman who has had a wonderful sex life with her husband believed she must be boringly normal, not

realising how rare it still is for healthy, straightforward
sexual talk between husband and wife. Not just of the
what goes where, right leg up a bit variety, but the whole
gamut of feelings and desires, so that one partner is in
touch and aware of the other's desires – and lack of desire.

Lack of desire in the husband, through age or health
problems, was accepted in a philosophical way by many
wives, some of whom were only too glad to be finished
with sex and who can blame them if they had never felt
pleasure, but only a regular duty?

The youngest woman I interviewed, still in her forties,
had been married twice and had only found sexual
happiness with her second husband. Raised by a repressive mother who believed sex was unpleasant, dirty and
not to be talked about, she still finds difficulty in coming to
terms with her sexuality. But she has forced herself to talk
to her children about sex, although it has been difficult
and embarrassing. She was determined that her daughter
would be well informed so that she would not suffer in the
same way.

Menopause brought general relief, women no longer
had to worry about pregnancy. Several mentioned that
they were scared stiff that they might be pregnant when
they first stopped having periods – one remembered her
mother getting pregnant around the time of her menopause. The freedom from pregnancy helped some women
find sexual pleasure for the first time and most women
reported enhanced sexual feelings. Fantasy seemed to
play an important part in menopause, many women
having sexual fantasies about men at work or strangers
on the bus.

Menopause was often a time when marriages seemed to
fail, leaving women to embark on new relationships. The
troubles that had built up in a marriage seemed to reach
crisis point at menopause. This was often put down to
mood changes by the women themselves, though it may

be that they were seeing the relationship clearly for the first time. Menopause shook things up and women had to think about themselves as women, sometimes for the first time in many years, and it often gave them the impetus for change.

As menopause could be a time when women found themselves on their own, through divorce or death, how did they adapt to their new lives as single women? Did they put up the barricades and heave a sigh of relief, or did they go out there again looking for new partners?

And what of their attitude towards the younger generations? I found them surprisingly liberal, delighted that their children and grandchildren had a better chance of sexual happiness and closer marriages. Most were firmly of the belief that marriage should be worked at, and worked at harder than many young people seem prepared to do, but that if it didn't work out then separation was the best option.

When I think of the woman who has been married for more than forty years with no sexual pleasure, her husband insisting that sex should stop at menopause, since it was for the procreation of children and not for pleasure; when I listen to her saying, without bitterness, that she didn't mind, but would have liked a token of affection or a cuddle in more than forty years of marriage, then I think we should all be made to take an A level in relationships and sexuality.

Katherine

Fifty-three. She is attractive and fashionably dressed. She is beginning to acknowledge difficulties in her marriage.

I would say possibly, most of the time, I have been disappointed with sex in our marriage. At the beginning being very amateur, neither of us having had much experience, we were rather fumbling away. It's partly my fault and I'm beginning to realise that and take matters into my own hands more and presumably that will improve things, hopefully. Either do that or split us up I think. It's curious, maybe I realise I've been disappointed and have just shut off where he is concerned. I suppose I ought to do something about it before it goes on too long.

My husband has not got enough work at the moment, so the roles have reversed quite extraordinarily in the last couple of years. It's taken a couple of years for him to get to the stage where he will now take over the washing and stuff – he hasn't got to the ironing yet, but that may come.

He's become rather uncertain about things. He watches me get dressed in the morning and says things like, 'What are you doing today? Why are you getting dressed up? Oh, that's a pretty bra', so there's a feeling of unease there that I might be inclined to stray and that would devastate him. He has always been very possessive and having had me for two-thirds of our marriage at his beck and call, tied to the house, has made him complacent and now it's changed. Also he's lost his identity with not working.

I answer back now, whereas before I didn't, simply because I didn't want any trouble. He is a very nice man, he's a very complex man, he's intellectually very bright and can run rings round me in arguments and discussions, so very often I've backed off having a discussion because I know I'm going to lose.

I would be a very peculiar person if I hadn't changed because almost by accident I have done pretty well in a late career start. I had children at twenty and then twenty-two and also we were living abroad and so I couldn't work. So it's really been very liberating for me, almost too late, and I'm enjoying every minute of it.

I call the shots a lot more in our sexual relationship,

saying no if I don't want to. I don't initiate yet, although possibly the way I behave initiates, but certainly if I don't want to I don't and that's it and I'm not so scared of hurting as I used to be. The dreadful thing is I'm not keen with my husband – there's an awful lot of sameness about one person after thirty-four years and the ability to surprise has gone. We could actually freshen it up, but we'd have to do some pretty funny things and I think neither of us wants to suggest something that might be considered a bit peculiar.

I do fantasise about sex, so I must still be interested in it. I do find myself dreaming about sex sometimes, invariably with my husband Paul. Once it was a colleague and that was very embarrassing because I don't actually fancy him at all and it's very funny because you have to face them the next day and hope they can't read your dreams!

I adore my husband. You know how sometimes you look at some people and you think, 'Poor things, they've been together for sixty years and they don't like each other very much'. I don't want that to happen to us, I want us to be good with each other, so working towards that, this is probably part of it.

Halfway through our interview Katherine suddenly sat bolt upright in her chair and told me that she had only just realised, in talking to me, that she had never had a very good sex life with her husband. We paused and looked at each other. It was one of those moments that makes you hold your breath as an interviewer; you know this is important and you don't want that fragile moment of trust to be lost. She went on to analyse the reasons and the way that the power relationship had changed between them. I was anxious at the end of the interview that we shouldn't just leave things hanging – I felt a responsibility to her, having elicited this insight. We talked through the various options open to her like counselling and she was clear that she needed to talk things through with Paul, although she also knew that that would be the most difficult part. She acknowledged her strong sexual desire, through dreams and fantasies and it became clear as we talked that some action was imperative.

Brenda

Fifty-four. Her face lights up when she talks about her husband. She resisted the idea she was going through menopause, even denying classic symptoms like hot flushes.

Menopause has made me more sexual. How often we have sex varies, two or three times a week on average and then I go without for a couple of weeks and it's really good. It varies so much from real lust to gentleness and that's what I find so great.

Me and my husband, we had a joke. I said you've got to go through two years without periods before you actually know and 1993 is going to be the turning point in our sexual relationship. 1993, yes! And it has been a turning point, it's really been good. It's partly knowing you can't get pregnant, and not using condoms is a real freedom. But freedom from pregnancy has brought its own problems; sometimes I feel that I could have sex, but do I want to?

My expectations are different from when we were first married. We never had sex before we were married. I didn't expect anything, he hadn't slept with anyone before either, or so he tells me, and I believe him. It was quite exploratory and I suppose I did quite a lot of the work. We weren't embarrassed, well, a bit initially, but we were both totally inexperienced.

Menopause has been negative for me physically, but my sex life is better. But I always think that's in my mind anyway – wanting sex or not wanting sex. Physically I felt it, but mentally I suppose I see things slightly clearer. There's no encumbrances.

Sex has got better over the years. Quite a big turning

point for us was that we bought a caravan by the seaside. We used to go there at weekends and it felt raunchy, it felt holidayish, and there was no phone. The other week we were going to meet some friends in the evening, from the caravan opposite. It was Saturday afternoon, we were in the shower and had it in the shower and it was lovely – of course we pulled the blind down. The neighbours knocked on the door and I just had this towel on. She felt embarrassed and we looked at one another and she said what have you two been up to!

We went through a phase, when the children were teenagers, when he said should we do something different. We got these videos out and I didn't like that at all. I'm going back years when they first came out. Gymslips and cucumbers – it was really naughty stuff and I didn't like it because I didn't know people did that. I don't like videos. I don't mind if he watches them, but my assumption is that they probably go too far. He said to me the other night, did I want to watch it? I said no and would I be surprised now at what they get up to, he said yes. I said would I like it and he said no. He knows where the limits are.

I think our relationship has grown. I've more or less said it's OK to do things that I felt before were not OK. We went through a phase when the children were still at home that when we had sex I was very conscious that they were in the house and I didn't feel free. Though I missed my eldest daughter terribly, there's much more freedom now. The day they left I shouted out to my husband, 'Yes! Yes!' [*she punches the air in a football victory salute*]. I could shout, I could do what I liked.

Menopause affected sex in so much as I was waking up two or three times in the night. You know you've got to get up at six o'clock to go to to work and I found that restricting. Your sleep was disturbed and if you had sex – the sheer fatigue.

It's mutual who decides to have sex. I can sort of sense . . . he gives me vibes and then very often it is left to me. He's quite a gentle man, and we talk to each other a lot during sex, saying do this or do that. The only thing I find difficult is sometimes he says, 'talk to me sexy or dirty', and I think 'oh dear'. That I find quite difficult.

We are compatible, but you need to work at it too. When I had my first baby, it was such a shock to me and my body, I didn't want anything to do with sex for a long time, nearly a year. I thought if you were breast feeding, you don't do it, yet he stayed with me. I suppose I don't forget those sorts of things.

And then he's had a major operation. The year before last he was in hospital, in intensive care for a long time and one of the first questions we asked was about sex. It was about four months that he was off work and then he went for a check-up and he wouldn't ask. So I asked and the doctor said it's fine as long as I'm on top and do all the work, and I said well that's nothing changed then, jokingly!

I work at being a bit interesting. We made love on the stairs once, and I was on the phone to somebody and her name was Mary Jones so now if we want to do anything, like when he was in hospital, I sent him a card and I signed it 'from Mary Jones' and everyone said who's Mary Jones! That's our little secret if you like. But normally, I say 'seen Mary?' and it's a sort of joke, like a codeword! It sometimes just happens or I suddenly wear something different that gives a signal. We're not embarrassed with each other – not long ago I said 'I'm supposed to have a G-spot somewhere, where is it?' I mean I haven't got a clue!

At one time I was just happy for him to get the pleasure, that was very important. I felt that was mega-important, he had a full-time job, he needed me and also, as he was in sales, I felt that there might be a bit of competition out there and I felt I had to make a few challenges. But I don't feel that so much anymore. It changed when I got my job, I felt that I was more of an equal.

Brenda had me roaring with laughter at her tales of sexual antics with her husband! She seemed a little embarrassed, asking me several times whether she might be too boring and ordinary to be interesting for this book. But it struck me that she was the very opposite – someone who had managed to make the sexual part of her marriage work and keep on working, despite both of them being inexperienced when first married. When she spoke of her husband she smiled, with a naughty glint in her eye, and she was obviously still delighted with him. The contrast with Katherine, who spoke fondly of her partner but who had clearly lost the sexual magic, was all the more striking. It made me wonder what it was, exactly, that made a marriage sexually compatible. Brenda's experience suggests that good humour, tolerance and strong communication must be three key factors.

Marjorie

Seventy-six. She is divorced after many years of marriage. She confounds all the stereotypes about older women and sexuality and takes great pleasure in doing so.

People tend to believe that before the sixties there was no sex, nobody ever did anything, and there were no dirty jokes. They should have gone through the fucking war and the fucking war before that!

During my married life I was very keen on sex, I thought it was wonderful. If we'd had sliced bread when I got married or when I first went into these things, I'd have said it was the nicest thing since. I don't think that was unusual in my generation, but people didn't talk about it out loud in case somebody else heard.

I wasn't a virgin when I got married so I knew what to expect – well I knew what I hoped! I hoped for a good time. I'd had a good sex life beforehand, well quite comfortable, you can put it that way.

No problem with contraception, and that's another thing that really annoys me. I grew up in what I call 'the CC' culture – cigarettes and condoms. My family all smoked; my father smoked, my mother smoked, my aunt smoked, everybody smoked, in the cinema, everywhere. Now similarly, people think there was no birth control. There's been birth control for years and years if people just bothered to find out about it. I would never have sex without a condom, and the reason for that was very simple; in my day we didn't have any antibiotics and although we didn't have AIDS, we did have syphilis, which was just as much a scourge in its way. I said this when I was quite young and I repeat it now, that I saw no reason whatever to be used as a sideline to a male urinal.

People of your generation assume that nobody knew anything, or that we never had sex before we got married. It isn't true. Read any decent literature, or perhaps that isn't the right word, read any literature of the period, it's just that it was done more discreetly. We were all the same, all my friends, and there was no problem.

I married my husband because I liked him best. Why did I get married when I disapprove of the process intensely and always have done? There were twelve in my mother's family, five in my father's family and nearly all the marriages came horribly unstuck, and I thought there is no way I am going to do that. Because if people love each other they will stay together without being tied in knots. If you tie them up in knots the chances are they will want to break the knots. It doesn't seem to me to be a very good idea.

I got married for a very different reason, not the traditional one – bombs, the blitz, and who picks up the pieces? If you have a blitz and a couple of pretty bad nights and you're both in the air raid shelters and if either one of us had been hit, the other one couldn't even pick up the pieces. Not legally. It concentrates the mind wonderfully, a good bomb.

We had a very open marriage and this worked fine. There were no problems of that sort at all. The thing that split us was something I can't understand and I've given up puzzling about it now – everyone who knows us is the same about this. He became a total alcoholic and in the end I couldn't cope with that. Because he who had loved animals so much, he threatened to break the dog's back with a pair of fire irons and that was it, so I threw him out. I was about fifty-four.

I divorced my husband and during that period I was a very good girl indeed – I couldn't afford to be otherwise and I didn't want to be otherwise. I was fed up with the whole bloody world of men to be honest, too much trouble. I didn't want anybody or anything, I just wanted to lick my wounds, because I had been torn sideways, upwards, downwards to make that marriage work.

I was getting knocked about too. The reason I was getting knocked about was not because I'm a coward or because I can't hit back, I was quite agile in those days and I used to pack a good punch; I used to be able to punch my weight quite well if I needed to. But simply that he had had a heart attack a good many years previously and after that, if he didn't get his own way entirely he'd say you're trying to cause me a heart attack. I had a horrible idea that he was trying to goad me into hitting him, so he could say that I had hit a sick man. That would put right on his side and I was not going to do that. I never hit him, I never touched him, but I became as good as Nigel Benn at bobbing and weaving. Not quite because I got some bruises and loose teeth and a few odds and ends like that and then I thought 'Fucking hell, I'm not going to put up with this any more. This is not on chum'.

After menopause, I did have an active sex life for a while, but then I really had too much to do. Also there was all this talk about AIDS and I was getting older, obviously, and I think it was Voltaire who said, sadly desirability dies before desire. I would never make a fool of myself deliberately, I may do it unconsciously. I have old friends who come and see me for a week and we're still very good, old friends and if we get together for a little bit, well that's our business.

I don't think sexual compatibility is chance. I think there's a certain chemistry – chemistry of attraction – and if there's a good attraction, then you're quite willing to spend an evening experimenting and adjusting and getting a good result.

It was good sleeping with the same person all that time, as long as the results were good. Look, you don't expect to have a raving orgasm every time, because that just does not happen, but there are other things to sex and other ways of achieving your results than bump, bump, bump and grind, grind, grind. I've tried most things but I do draw the line at anal sex or anything like that. I think that is for other people. It isn't all about orgasm, that's another thing about your generation, you're obsessed with orgasm; you can have lots of fun, there are lots of things you can do without being too kinky or going into any of the more esoteric forms.

Marjorie took great relish in confounding my preconceptions about older women and sex. She had been sexually active before marriage, had enjoyed sex very much with her husband and had agreed to an open marriage with him. She maintained that many women were just as sexually free in their twenties and thirties as the present generation, the difference was they didn't talk about it. And that women were very sexually active during the war. Marjorie's marriage broke up during her menopause when the violence and alcoholism of her husband became too much, but I wondered how far the menopause itself was responsible.

Rose

Eighty-four. Although only eight years older than Marjorie, Rose belongs to a different generation and class, which gave her a completely different outlook on sex.

Nature made the man feel that he wanted to make love, but if you were the woman, you didn't know whether you did or you didn't because there was no fondling – they didn't give you no cuddling. Really they should have done as they do now. But it was like some of these foreign countries, you were there, so that when the man came home, you had to do his bidding and it wasn't in love, it was just to satisfy him.

My husband, he was four years older than me and like everyone else, if it came to him that he felt he wanted sex, he used to kind of get hold of me and cuddle me, but not the way it is today. There's books about everything today. In the past, a woman never really and truly enjoyed sex, I don't think she did. When you got married, you had to do it, whether you wanted to or not. But there was no cuddling, no comfort like that, they were all the same.

My husband never drank much because he was always ill and couldn't afford it. But men would come home from public houses of a Sunday, they'd have to carve the meat and no one must dare interfere – most men were like that – then after that, he'd send the children off to Sunday school or somewhere else and his wife would have to follow him upstairs for him to have sex with her. There was no love. Now, it's as it should have been years ago. It's sad, because the women really, I suppose, would have liked to have had sex, and then men were as ignorant as the women. It was a thing you were brought up to keep secret, it was a secret thing.

I was married in April 1924 and he died twenty-five years ago. He gave me a card for our anniversary and died

two days later. We got on well, but like everybody else we
had our quarrels. He had such a lot of bad health when
the boys were young. I was very patient, it's your husband
for better or for worse and I looked after him the best I
could. I went to work, I used to always go to work,
cleaning in a pub for a few hours at eight pence an
hour. Then I worked at the water board, cleaning for
two hours and a quarter; go to work about quarter to six,
then I used to get the boys off to school, then go back in
the evening and Saturday morning and Saturday afternoon.

My mother was most secretive when it come to anything about sex. I always remember what she said to me;
she said, 'Now Rose', when I had my periods start, 'there's
the pieces of cloth, fold them up and stitch them up. You
have to put them on, then you wash them'. That was all
she said, nothing about sex.

The first thing I remember learning about sex, I was on
the way to school. There was a shop with postcards and
there was a big card of a field. There were cabbages
growing and babies were gradually growing as well – the
heads were growing and the arms were growing. And
there was a man and a lady, dressed in the old-fashioned
suit and costume. The man had a stick and he was
pointing to one he thought he would like when they
were fully grown. That is really where I thought babies
came from!

My husband was a pretty good-looking man. I was
eighteen when I got married. I was happy in marriage, he
was quite friendly and nice with me, but you didn't get the
loving when he came home, like you see today, all that
fondness. They thought it was a bit stupid, a bit nancyish.
The feeling was if you did that, people would look at you
and think you were a bit stupid. Really, if they'd had done
that years ago, shown their feelings, it would have relaxed
the woman. If you were to talk about your sexual feelings

in those days, they'd think you were very bad. It wasn't recognised.

Rose is an affectionate, warm woman, who kisses me on the cheek when I leave. I feel terribly sad that she has had no chance for a happy sexual life because of ignorance and lack of education in sexual matters. She didn't have access to information in the way someone like Marjorie did only a few years later – and that is as much a matter of the differences in class as anything else. She doesn't complain, but looks rather wistfully at her children and grandchildren. Nor does she blame her husband – that's just how things were in her time. She describes her marriage as happy, though her husband took no notice of her and was obviously a clumsy, ill-informed sexual partner. It makes me feel grateful that I live in a different time and place.

Annie

Fifty-six. She feels bitter about the failure of a long-term relationship.

I haven't been in that many actual relationships. I had my first lesbian relationship when I was at school, I was seventeen. I was dreadfully innocent and naïve, but it was a sexual relationship. She was a little bit older than me, I was in the year behind her. When she had taken her A levels, we were both going to leave school and go off and live in Switzerland because her father was going to get us a job there. So I left school before I had taken my A levels, I was all lined up to go to university but I left school and she immediately decided that she was heterosexual and got herself a boyfriend.

So there I was, with a few O levels and no job and a broken heart. For many years after that I lived at home with my mother, alone of course. I was celibate for many years because I could not fancy boys. I lived in a very boring suburb of London where in order to find boys you had to join the church youth club, there was no other way.

So I had this sexless life until I had quite a bad nervous breakdown when I was twenty-six. I went into hospital for five months, and I met this woman who had been extremely heterosexual, if I can put it that way; she had had more boyfriends and more sex than I had had hot dinners. I guess basically I was seduced by her, it was the one thing she hadn't done. She was a bit younger than me. We had what I would call my first grown-up affair. I was then twenty-seven and that lasted off and on for about three years. She wouldn't actually live with me – we were under the same roof and had rooms in the same house – she was frightened of her sexuality and what was happening to her, and she didn't like to admit it even to herself, although she does now.

Then followed a period of celibacy. I tried, I did my best to be heterosexual, it was like taking medicine! I slept with men, not very many; it wasn't so much the sex that was so awful – to a certain extent sex can be a bit mechanical, like twiddle a knob and XYZ happens – but there was no emotional content to it at all. And I didn't actually want to hurt anybody and I started feeling bad about it. I started feeling as if I was experimenting on men.

They made the first move, I didn't have to do anything. It was curiosity – I thought I didn't want to go to my grave a technical virgin. And it was the loneliness of living in a bedsitter, thinking I was the only lesbian for several hundred miles. I felt I'd really got to try and be heterosexual or I was going to be on my own forever. I thought, 'Everybody else does it', but it didn't work. What was awful was that afterwards I didn't want to have anything to do with them, and in the morning I'd want them to push off, have this piece of toast and go! You can't do that can you? But that's what I wanted! There was no cuddliness or warmth or emotional thing there at all.

I'm talking about 1966–67. There was no lesbian line, so where did I go? I'd left home by then and was living in a flat. I didn't know any lesbians. I believe there was one club running then, in Chelsea, but I didn't know where it was. If I'd known where it was, I'd have been too frightened to go there, so what could I do? I was lonely and I was young and I was a sexual person then. So I tried my luck with men, but it didn't work, after a bit I thought this isn't doing anybody any good, but then somebody else came into my life.

I'd got used to living by myself by then, I'd been on my own for about four years. She wanted to marry me, if I can put it that way. We shared a mortgage, shared a car, shared two cats, the usual stuff. Then, after I'd lived with her for eight years, she decided she'd got fed up with me, exchanged me for a new model. That was awful! I lost my house, which is why I'm living in a housing association flat. I have no car, I have no partner. I got custody of the cats and the cooker. It was just as bad as any heterosexual marriage that breaks up, with all the acrimony.

I was forty-eight when she buggered off. I wasn't expecting it, we hadn't rowed; she'd done it once before, gone off and had an affair with somebody and I'd taken her back and she just went and did it again. I guess she was fed up with me. I could see why, because our relationship hadn't been sexual for a long time and that was mainly down to me.

It started to fail as soon as we started to live together. I felt as if I was being taken over and I was, down to things like the colour of the wallpaper. She would come in and say, 'Mmm, I think we'll do this room orange', and I would say 'Wait a minute, there are two people living in this house', and she would look quite shocked. It seemed to me, the only place I could hold on to myself was in bed and I could say no there and I did. In that way you could say it was my fault, but it's much more complicated than that.

Sexual compatibility is something that's very difficult to work at; I think it is mainly chance. Having said that, you can know a person for a while and then fancy them, but basically I think it happens rather quickly, usually. You can work at making sex better, once you've started having sex, but I think that initial attraction has to do with magnetism and eye contact and all sorts of imponderables that we don't know about.

The awful thing is, I fancy heterosexual women much more than lesbians. I can't really say why it is, maybe it's the unattainable, partly, and to fall for someone who is out of reach is much safer than someone who's available.

Again Annie made me feel how much better it is to be living here and now. It seems tragic that she tried to have relationships with men in order to feel 'normal' and like everyone else, when her whole sexual orientation is clearly gay. Annie doesn't seem to expect much from life – she's setting herself up for failure by admitting to fancying heterosexual women who she knows probably won't want a relationship with her. It seems like a mirror image of her early behaviour, when she was trying to sleep with men.

Elizabeth

Seventy-seven. She belongs to the generation that believes you have to make the best of things, no matter what. She has remained remarkably cheerful, despite a difficult marriage.

Unfortunately my husband has never been particularly interested in sex. He's a very Victorian type who thinks that sex is for procreation and not enjoyment. He felt a bit guilty if he enjoyed sex and quite honestly once my periods stopped, he lost interest completely.

I'm certain sex was never discussed in his household at all! And of course, it was probably partly my fault too, because you see my generation, we never made the advances. It wasn't the thing to do, you left it to the man and of course if the man didn't make them well of course that was that! [*She laughs*] It's very different now I know!

You found out about sex from your friends. I was rather fortunate because I worked in the Civil Service and my woman supervisor was a very forward-thinking person. I suppose that nowadays she would be called a lesbian, but we never thought of such things in those days! But she did introduce me to Marie Stopes and talked about sex. That was a revelation to me.

I remember when I went out with a boy, I suppose I was fourteen or fifteen and I was absolutely horrified when he put my hand on his penis and I could feel this hard line! I went home as quickly as I could, I didn't know what it was you see, despite the fact that I had brothers. That was the incredible thing.

When I was married the first time, we'd been friends for quite a long time. There again it wasn't terribly physical, but intellectually we were great friends. Then of course the war came and he was killed and that was that. My first two children are his children. I was young enough then to miss the physical side, not terribly, but there were times when I would have liked to have had a cuddle.

When the children were old enough to go to school, I went to work and met my present husband at work. That was the amazing thing, he was quite happy taking on two children. We were in our thirties then. Then again, he was an intellectual; it sounds silly doesn't it, but I always needed somebody I could talk to, discuss things with. We used to have long discussions about all kinds of things and I suppose there was a certain amount of physical attraction, but it wasn't overwhelming in any way.

It's very different from today, this business that you see on television – I have never experienced emotions like that at all! I think a bit more physical business would have been better, it would have been a warmer relationship. I think women do want to be cuddled – it wasn't so much the sexual act, but I would have loved him to have put his arms round me and just cuddled me and I think that is what women do need. Also they desperately do need to feel wanted. Men are not very good at that, not at all.

Nowadays people would go for counselling, but it would have never have occurred to me. I have thought recently that he needed help, but I never thought so when we were younger, I just accepted him. He was in his thirties when we got married and he had had very, very few female friends prior to that.

Until we married we had no physical relationship; he was very strict about that, we both were really. Quite honestly, I decided eventually that the reason he married me was because his mother was getting very old and he knew that he was going to need a housekeeper one day. Also he did want to have a family. Fortunately I don't need an awful lot of sex, but I do need warmth and kindness.

My husband's become disabled. Of course it's meant he's had to give up his car. I naturally have to do a lot for him, but he hates it, he almost physically pushes me away. And he's never kind and loving about it at all. It is difficult and if the physical relationship had continued, it would have helped I'm sure. I would love to be able to put my arm round him and cuddle him a bit but he would just push me away, he almost builds a wall round himself, it's terrible.

Listening to Elizabeth made me angry. How could a man have treated this warm, affectionate, attractive woman so coldly? And how did she put up with it for all these years without protest? She had coped with the death of her first husband in war, believing, like many of her generation, that these things happened and you had to get on with life. What shocked me most was that she had never protested, all those long, cold years of married life, nor made demands when he had decided, unilaterally, to give up sex when she went through menopause.

Clare

Fifty-six. Younger women's lives can be complicated too. Clare's husband is a vicar. Loyalty is a strong factor in her marriage.

I was twenty when I first got married. I'd never lived away from home, I'd never been to college or anything like that. I moved straight into a house and marriage from my parent's home. It was quite a shock, I can remember my husband went off to work and I just sat and cried and thought what am I supposed to do in this new house and what am I?

He was super, physically, my first husband. I did know about sex, though when I met Bill I was a virgin. He had obviously had experience, but he was super with me. We had a child straight away. We did love each other and had a good relationship to start with. I was very young and then I grew up and we grew apart. It was mutual – the children were thirteen and nine we when split up. I lived on my own for a while and we separated amicably. I have to say now that we didn't make very much effort at trying to get our relationship together again. The split appeared to come from me, but looking back now, it was mutual.

My first husband is a strong, determined person and he said, 'Right this is it'. He took himself off and he bought himself a home. There were no financial worries at all and he built up a new social life, married a widow, a very nice lady and he's been very happy. He never harassed me or blamed me or anything like that, he started a new life and that was that. I see him through the children at christenings, weddings, that sort of thing, perhaps at Christmas. It's not difficult, he's probably quite fond of me, we had a very amicable divorce.

I met Stephen quite soon afterwards, but he was married at the time. It was very difficult. When we met, I knew this was someone I wanted to be with. We met socially at a friend's house, at a dinner party. It was very hard for him because of his profession, he had children at boarding school, there were the financial pressures, and he felt very guilty over the whole thing, but he wasn't happy with his wife. So it was a long process, he did swing from one to the other and then he did separate and divorce but it was very hard for us both. He still feels guilt now. We were married about six years after we met.

We were hugely attracted to each other and yet I have to say it wasn't easy. I did wonder what on earth I was doing, that maybe it was better not to stay with him, that maybe it was better to stay on my own, but we did love each other.

I love him and we are still together. It's been extremely difficult, he's had a lot of problems, but I guess I have too. Things haven't been easy. He had a drinking problem brought on, or accentuated, by his problems and he lost several jobs and went abroad to work.

He's always been a super, gentle, kind person. He's a dear, he's lovely. We've been married sixteen years. I did have someone to compare with and I think Stephen will always have problems feeling guilty, I really do, and that did affect our marriage. And yet physically we are very attracted. Nowadays people are more open about these things, we should have had help and counselling. But again it is very difficult for Stephen because he thinks he should know the answers. He's great at listening to everybody else, he's super, but when it comes to himself that is entirely different. How can he own up to weaknesses?

I can never say that our sexual relationship was good. It is difficult to talk about it to him, it's very difficult. He just gets desperately upset and bottles it all up. And obviously when you're drinking, you lose all sexual drive altogether.

I think of myself as quite a sexual person, it has been hard, having had one marriage with good sex and then going into another marriage where sex was a problem. I certainly didn't want sex to go by the board, I wanted to work at it. We have got a good relationship, we love each other but it isn't a strong physical relationship. I do feel we have missed out on a certain closeness that we could have had. He is quite affectionate, and we cuddle and hug. Sexuality can be expressed in other ways and so I try to shut my mind to things. I keep very busy and I accept it; not everybody goes through life having a good sexual relationship.

I have often been tempted to leave, often, then I just think I can't, certainly now he's had this serious heart attack I can't; probably I'm a bit resentful of that. I'd be frightened of a life without him, very frightened, because he's a prop for me, because my energies are directed towards looking after him. Often I think, 'I would like to be out of this', but then I think, 'How would I cope and what would I do?' I've thought about this a lot; basically I'm a bit of a coward and don't know what life I would be going to. I'm not strong enough to think, 'Right, I will go and make a new life'. I think I've got cold feet.

Clare's second marriage and her acceptance of their sexual difficulties shows how wrong our assumptions often are about how relationships work. She gave up her first husband with whom sex worked well. Her second husband felt such enormous guilt at leaving his wife that it has left a sexual cloud over the marriage. And the fact that he is in a caring profession has enabled him to look

*after others and sort out their problems, but left him unable to ask
for help himself. Yet, despite the temptation to leave, this attractive,
still young woman has chosen not to have affairs or leave altogether,
but to stay.*

Caroline

*Seventy-three. Her marriage difficulties highlight the ignorance of
the medical profession in dealing with marital problems in the past.*

My present husband and I married in 1945. We'd known
one another for about five years – we'd been up at
university together – and I was just twenty-five. We
were married just before the end of the war and we both
went on working. Then I produced identical twin daughters, so I gave up work.

We parted after about eighteen years of marriage; it
was all a very sad and difficult time. After a year or two,
we both remarried and neither marriage was a success
really because we should never have parted. He and his
wife eventually separated and my husband died and in the
course of time, we came together again and we've been
together for about ten years.

My mother never talked to me about sex, people didn't
in those days. I often look back on her life and conjecture
what sort of life it was. My father had psoriasis very badly,
which made him irritable. He was the kindest of men but I
don't think he was terribly easy to live with. You always
assume your marriage will be much like your parents.

I did know about sex when I got married. Mostly what
I learnt, I learnt from my husband, and when I was at
school we used to devour books which hinted at the 'Great
Event'! And we conjectured what it was all about, but
premarital sex didn't really go on at all. My father would
have been absolutely horrified. Michael and I both loved
each other and he was understanding and gentle, and it

wasn't any sort of shock at all, it was enjoyable. We've had a good physical relationship on the whole.

Later on, when our marriage ran into trouble, we went to see a doctor, a psychiatrist and he said, 'I can put everything right; in six months' time, you'll be sending me a thank-you card'. He put us both on a course of LSD. I went up to the clinic one week and he went up the next, so we each had it once a fornight for about eighteen months, a long gruesome business. It would last all day and then about tea time, whoever hadn't had it would fetch the other in the car.

It was a peculiar experience. Once you'd had it, you got the feeling that you must go the next week. Actually I used to look forward to going because it wasn't unpleasant all the time. You had an injection, lay on the bed, then it would begin to work and you would get a really awful feeling, ghastly! Then you had this other stuff, called ritalin, that was injected. That really made the LSD work and you felt a sense of peace. You could lie back and relax and go right into whatever it was that was coming up in your mind. The idea was that it would liberate whatever it was that was causing problems in our marriage. Then we were supposed to talk it through with the doctor, but they didn't do that nearly enough in my opinion. If we'd had really good counselling, it would have helped our marriage.

My experience was that I recollected my father having abused me a lot as a small child. Now I don't know whether this is actually true. To some extent, I think it's not impossible but I don't know, it's difficult to separate from the effects of the LSD. He certainly was a man who liked the girls. It was pretty shattering, that experience. My husband went through a bad time over it, in fact, that is what really caused the break-up of our marriage.

I regret it very much, it was an absolute disaster, we'd been married about eighteen years. My mother was very sad when I got divorced because in her day divorce didn't happen except in Hollywood! Even when we divorced, it wasn't anything like as common as it is now.

I was separated for two years, then met someone else. I was forty-six when I married my second husband, David, a friend of Michael's. He'd had a very difficult life. He was Polish by birth and spent all his youth in Germany. He was Jewish and had been thrown into a concentration camp and had a very bad time in Dachau. He did escape and came to England and joined the Special Operation Executive and went out again. He was very brave but he had had such a bad time, he was very scarred by it really. I fell for him, we had a very good sexual relationship, he was great fun, but very, very jealous and possessive.

I can remember the first night of our marriage, we were out having dinner and I was just watching some people at the next table. I suddenly realised he was getting very angry, so I asked him what the matter was, he said I was making eyes at the man at the next table!

We did spar a bit over our children. He had children by a former marriage and we had very different ways of bringing them up. It was very difficult, they were all teenagers, his as well as mine – he had four children who lived with his ex-wife. I felt that he allowed them much more licence than he would allow my children and yet he could be extremely kind, very amusing and witty; we had some good laughs with them.

Things like Christmas were difficult because he had the continental background and Christmas eve to him was the time to have the presents and meal and you know how traditional children are. My children didn't like that at all, Christmas Day was the day for them. So we had his children on Christmas eve. I used to dread Christmas!

My happiness with him, sexual happiness particularly, was feeling accepted again in that field. My husband had had this other woman for a couple of years and when you feel rejected, you don't feel attractive any more, you feel unwanted. With David, there was no doubt whatever that he wanted me and that was good, so the early part of our marriage we did have a very good sexual relationship. But as we settled down, I found the fact that his background was so different increasingly difficult. He'd been marvellously brave, but he'd been through experiences which just do affect you always. We can't imagine it at all. Our physical relationship diminished and he found that hard to take. I wasn't interested anymore because of all the difficulties.

We were married for eight years. We came to a point when I said we can't go on, we were both unhappy and I think I felt it more strongly than he did – I knew it was wrong. It just came suddenly, though he was being more and more difficult. It was Christmas eve and I had to go to work and that annoyed him as we were supposed to go over to his daughter. I got off work a bit early and went over there, but the door was locked. I thought they had gone for a stroll so I hung around for a bit. It was very cold and I suddenly thought, 'Blow me, I'm not hanging round here', so I went home. I rang two friends in the country and went to stay with them, they asked no questions. I stayed about three days and when I came home he was there and didn't ask any questions either and I thought 'Right, this is it, this is too ridiculous', so that was when I said it had better come to an end. Leaving was the difficult time. I waited until he had to go out on a business trip. It sounds awful, but I thought it was the only way to do it. I'd arranged for the furniture removal to come and I was very careful to take only the things that had belonged to my family and my first marriage. He came back and found I'd gone. He knew where I was and we met several times after that, b.. I knew it was the right thing to do, that was what gave me the courage to do it.

I was lucky that financially I could do it, because I was

earning quite a lot – it does make a difference. I'm sure women put up with more in the past because they had no choice. Although sometimes, if you can put up with it, things work out later on. Sex ceases to be so important and once that dies down, then the friendship side of marriage becomes more important. All our children had left home by then. He later had a heart attack and died at the airport, on the way to a concentration camp reunion.

Michael and I had never completely broken off all contact because of the children – he'd come down for their weddings, etc. – and whenever we met we knew the spark was still there. The thing that had parted us didn't seem to matter so much any more, after all those years. His wife was very dependent and extravagant and he didn't know how to leave her, he felt he couldn't do it. He'd become very addicted to alcohol, to such an extent that he was hardly able to do his work and then he retired. It took six years before I was able to persuade him that he needed help, but he went in the end and is completely cured.

I did have misgivings about getting back together, I certainly did, as we'd been separated for nineteen years. Whenever we met, I felt something still there but I threw myself into work and friends and other interests. I wasn't interested in other men, I'd had my fill by then! We had lunch together one day, when I happened to be on holiday near where he worked. He was in such a sad way and so obviously just dying to come back. It was about a week after that that they rang from work and more or less said he was on his way. I was clear that I wanted him back, I'd been on my own for eight years then. We got married again and resumed our life together, but not on a sexual basis at all.

Looking at my children's marriages and lives now and the things that go wrong, one tends to think perhaps that it's because of what happened and I have certainly been through a great deal of guilt about it all, but you can't live with guilt for the rest of your life.

Caroline should have been celebrating her golden wedding anniversary in 1995. The thought of this conventional, thoughtful woman being subjected to LSD injections once a fortnight for eighteen months, fills me with horror. It's astonishing that either of them managed to hang on to their sanity. Caroline stressed her belief that good counselling at the appropriate time might have saved that first marriage and the intervening difficult years. She's one of life's copers, who gets on with whatever is thrown at her, but she seems now, after menopause, to have achieved a happy balance in her life.

Alice

Sixty. She describes herself as a walking disaster area as far as relationships are concerned.

I've been led by my passionate nature. I regret that and the terrible thing is, both times I got married, I knew I was doing wrong but I didn't have the courage to turn round and say no. I didn't dare say no, in case nobody else would ever want me. The day I got married the first time, I realised it was wrong in the car going to church. The second time it was just before we moved in together, but I didn't want to lose my house.

We were married two and half years, then I met number two within a year of the break-up and we were married for twenty-five years. Now, I am living together with my first husband again, but we aren't married. When I met up again with my first husband, he showed me his bank statement in his pocket, very odd! I was taken in by him again – I should have stopped myself. I often wondered what he was doing – he was an absolute bastard – and whether he had changed. Of course when I met him again, I thought he'd changed totally, but had he buggery! Back to square one again.

All I've ever wanted in life is to have enough money. I'm very naïve and I just feel everything is going to be hunky dory if you've got enough money because it will make everything much easier.

My second husband was an absolute waster as well. I chose exactly the same men and they chose exactly the same as their mother. I would have loved to have had someone where I didn't have to worry about money all the time, how to pay the bills and where I could go on holiday a couple of times a year without the tremendous pressure to earn money.

I suppose fun attracts me and perhaps, on one level, knowing they are bad and wanting to change them or feeling you can change them.

When I married my first husband I was a virgin – in the fifties you didn't sleep with people before marriage, although I would have loved to. I've always had this sexual appetite. My father is still alive, my mother said he was active until a few years ago, when he had his prostate operation. I'm very much like him.

When I met my second husband he was ten years older than me, very much a man of the world, a very colourful character. Perhaps that's what I go for, people who are colourful. So sex with him was very exciting. In between them I had a grand passion with a musician, again that was all sexual; it was fantastic, it was great. He used to come home and sit sobbing at two in the morning after a bad performance and I'd take care of him and then we would go to bed and then he would go home. He was divorced.

With my second husband the sex petered out, as it does with everybody. It really was an intrusion, I just didn't want sex at all. I didn't want it with anyone else either. I can say, hand on heart, I never went with or looked at another man when I was married for the second time. I just lost interest. Then I met my first husband again before my second divorce, so I had the excitement there, in my early fifties, actually staying in a hotel! At first when I met up with him again, it was great – every stolen moment we were having sex, so in a way it was fantastic because I thought I can't get pregnant and here I am having sex and of course that has all worn off now. It made me feel freer and more relaxed about sex. I became very sexually active again at fifty-two, it was unexpected.

Anything you have to work at is an absolute sham. If you had to work at sex, that would be awful! It shouldn't be something that you have to think about. It horrifies me that all these books say, do it this way, do it that way, stick your leg up here!

Both men had always had loads of women; the first one cheated on his second wife like mad because he was very, very sexually active. Sex was great with them both. The first thing is that it must work sexually, nobody gets together with someone unless it is sex first, it's all passion and sex, that's what attracts you to each other. Great, I want to go to bed, can't eat, the stomach is churning, I want to go to bed with this man.

My sons tell me that their father wasn't faithful towards the end. My first husband wasn't faithful either – I don't think so. I put a detective on his tail and found an Irish girl, who had a baby, which he swears was not his, but of course he is such a sodding liar.

I wasn't attracted to my second husband any more, because he'd let me down. I'd had so many car boot sales, before there were car boot sales, it wasn't true. I was always having to bloody make do and mend, which I am now, and that affected the way I felt. I swear to you if there had been enough money and if I hadn't felt let down it would have been different.

I withdrew my favours because of being let down. I've

done this in the last couple of weeks with my present
partner. I don't want sex, I don't allow myself to be
propositioned, I push him away, turn over in bed. I've
been led by my passionate nature, rather than by my
head, definitely. I do regret it, I've had a good time but I
do regret it.

*Listening to Alice, I can't believe that this competent, capable
woman who seems so confident has followed such a disastrous path
in her sexual relationships. She described herself as a walking
disaster area. She had knowingly taken up with her first husband
again, expecting him to have changed. And although she can analyse
her mistakes and laugh about them ruefully, I get the feeling that if
another disaster area with panache and money were to walk through
the door, she would be first in the queue! It's love as social work,
taking someone and their problems on, despite one's better judgement. Her sexual appetite has not diminished but she seems to be
able to turn it on and off, like the gas, according to how pleased she
is with her partner.*

Madeleine

*Seventy-three. Her face shines with delight when she talks about her
marriage. Later I have coffee with them both and they are clearly in
harmony with each other.*

I've been married forty-six years gone, it's been wonderful, wonderful. I always feel I got rid of the horrible bits of
my life by the time I was twenty and then, you've been a
good girl, now you can start enjoying yourself! There's a
lot of joy, it's been wonderful for me, and so supportive.
    I don't think anything is chance, there is a purpose and
a plan. He's seven years older than I am and at one point I
thought he was far too serious. He gave me lectures about
different things and there I was, bored to the eyeballs! He
says he knew I was the one and he had to get across his

feelings about things. So there I was at eighteen, standing there thinking, 'Here he goes again'! But there was something about him. We did break up for a few weeks and then we just met by chance – or was it chance? – and that was it, back on again. The bond is clearly very strong between us.

My father left us when I was five, my mother struggled on, tried to commit suicide unsuccessfully and she died when I was eight. I was taken to live first of all with my grandmother, with my brother, and she really couldn't cope with two little children. Then I was taken to my aunt and very happily brought up, but almost a duty thing, so there wasn't affection shown and I had to learn that.

Really it was my husband who taught me to show affection and love. It's taken me years and years, but now I am very spontaneous and I do show it. My aunt didn't tell me about sex, she was very Victorian and strict. When she talked about periods coming, she said sometimes, instead of going to have a wee, it's blood that comes. That was it, that was all, nothing else!

I thought it was soft and silly to show affection. I did feel for people, but you didn't go and put your arm round them, it was all sloppy stuff. I met a man who is all demonstrative and slowly it warmed me up and took that shell off me, so now I am much more demonstrative.

I think the components of a good marriage are respect and doing for others as you hope to be done to. Respect – you give them their place and space. People now think they have a right to be happy and if they are not happy, whose fault is it? Theirs! *You* are not making *me* happy. Well, nobody makes you happy, it's inside you, you have to be happy inside. So it is knowing that it is not always going to be cloud nine, that there are going to be depressing times.

We support each other, complement each other in many ways. The physical side has been terrific, absolutely terrific until about ten years ago, when not only was there dryness but terrific pain. The doctor gave me pessaries but they haven't worked. We try now and again but it is just so painful that it's impossible. So we live on our memories of how great it was! Even now, Christopher says we don't need sex, so we cuddle, that's sexuality too. Sex is not necessarily intercourse, it's that loving and closeness and when you walk by, you touch them, just to show them you love them.

A happy sex life depends on the sex drive of the two partners. There's nothing worse than having a strong libido and finding there is frustration because of the other partner. That could really break up a marriage, but it's really difficult to find two people with the same level. Christopher has more drive than I have, but I love him for it, when you see someone with terrific energy in any job, I'm sure a high libido goes with that – it's an energy level.

When I got married, I didn't have any particular expectation of sex. I just thought I would enjoy it, everybody else seemed to be enjoying it! Fortunately I was never around these women who say 'Oh well, he's demanding', or 'He has his rights'! I never had that, that's what you gave up to have your roof and your food!

I had had sex before I got married – not very satisfactory! So I knew what to expect, but it was much better with Christopher. The first was a young man who really didn't know what he was doing and Christopher was a very sensitive lover always, it was very good.

People don't seem to discuss what they like and don't like. It's strange isn't it, that you can live with somebody all those years. You like them as a person, but not on the sexual side. You're missing out on a whole chunk of life, and it's the icing on the cake really.

Having a good partner is a good start to a good marriage, someone who supports you and really helps.

It's feeling that there is a helpmate there who is not out to score points from you and hurt you, so I have to pay back the same feelings to him.

Maybe people are looking for more, demanding more than the other person can give. I don't think there is 'a person', I think there is a type that you would be happy with, but it just needs a little extra to give it a zing. And if you do have a bad marriage, maybe this time round you are here to learn from a disastrous marriage. What is it teaching you, what can you learn from it? Unfortunately, so many people seem to marry again and they haven't brought any wisdom to that second marriage. Everything, even a disaster is a learning process.

So many women are disappointed. I think women read too many articles in magazines, you know, the man on the white charger whisking her off and so many of these young girls think that the wedding day is the culmination of dreams – that's just the start of the drudgery! I think we are fed wrong expectations.

Madeleine radiated happiness. While she was making coffee, her husband popped his head round the door and said he knew he was not really supposed to be talking to me, but he'd entertain me while the coffee was brewing. He seemed completely at ease with himself, and me, and we chatted happily for ten minutes. He was the only husband of the whole group to appear and be quite happy about what was going on. When I asked Madeleine what her secret was, she giggled and said that if she knew, she would bottle it and make a fortune. There was an easiness between them, a feeling of harmony and peace that made me reluctant to leave. Yet they were not complacent, they clearly still worked hard at making it successful.

Mavis

Seventy-three. She is a widow who had a happy marriage.

I've been married twice, I was married during the war but that didn't work out – it was one of those things – so then I married again. My second husband died sixteen years ago. I've been on my own since then.

No one talked about sex a great deal. As a young woman, I was very disappointed in sex; my first partner was very inexperienced. For that reason I think it might be a good idea for people to live together before they get married, to get to know someone sexually. But in those days you didn't.

As I've got older, my sexuality is much better. With my second husband I was more mature and had a different attitude towards it, we were more liberated. We had more practice, as you're growing older and you've been with someone for a while, you get to know them and know what they like and they know what you like, so obviously it's going to be better.

I think a longer relationship is better than a one-night stand from the sexual point of view, you've got to know someone really well to enjoy it. We were married thirty-four years. You like different things as you get older and you are quite happy to talk about it and say 'I don't like that, don't let's do that, let's maybe do something else'.

Touch is important. And so many relationships fail because people don't talk, or they can't talk, or they don't want to talk. If you can say this is what is wrong and this is why I don't want to sleep with you, or want you to touch me, or say I don't like what you're doing to me, can we do something else, then you build up good lines of communication. It might not always work but often it does, you have to try.

Mavis is matter of fact about her relationships. She looks fifteen years younger than her age. She talks glowingly of her second husband and shows that it is not just the younger generation who know how to talk about sex to their partners. I can't help

*contrasting her with Rose, Alice and Elizabeth who have had
such different expectations and experiences. Is it chance, or what you
are willing to put up with in life? Mavis divorced her first husband
and one senses that she would not have tolerated the behaviour that
Alice and Elizabeth have.*

Florrie

*Eighty-four. She has been married twice and now has a live-in
boyfriend. She has always liked the company of men.*

When I got married I was a virgin. I wasn't innocent, I'd
had boyfriends but you were supposed to wait because of
the neighbours! It seems daft now, be home at ten o'clock
because you'd got to watch the neighbours, oh yes, it was
always the neighbours when I was young. I wasn't really
tempted, I was a bit of a tomboy, much preferred boys to
girls. I loved running.

I'd known this boy for years and we got engaged when I
was twenty-one but he got a job in Scotland and we broke
it off. He wrote and said did I mind if he took out his
landlady's daughter? So I thought, 'if that is how you feel'
and I broke it off. I was very upset but didn't let him think
I was. You can't have two people, can you? I was very
upset for a long time. That was my real experience of boys.
I think the fact that we hadn't slept together made it
easier for him to break away.

I used to go dancing and my husband liked me. He was
much older than me – he'd been in the First World War –
he was forty and I was twenty-four, so there was quite a
big age gap. But he was a very nice person, adoring, too
much so really! He did the cooking and cleaning – a nice
man.

He was sexually experienced. I wasn't marvellously in
love with him, that's why I didn't have any children
probably. We were married twelve years. He didn't want

children, he was terrified of my dying, he'd lost one wife through heart disease. He didn't want to risk it so he used condoms. I didn't mind.

I never enjoyed sex. We just thought it was there and something you had to do, no violent feelings at all! My generation knew nothing, my mother had never told me anything abut sex, that sort of thing didn't happen, it just didn't happen. It was a bit of a shock, but you accept it because you like the person. I think lots of people of my generation felt like that.

I never knew there was anything like a girl having a reaction, you know like an orgasm, not until a friend of mine was speaking to me and said that she had never had an orgasm (she didn't call it that because we didn't even know what it was it called!) until her husband felt sorry for her and helped her, put his finger up her. 'Ooh,' she said, 'it was marvellous. Have you had one?'

I didn't know anything about that until I got married the second time. You did it for his sake, there was no idea that you had any pleasure at all. And if you had children as well that must have been very upsetting I should think, no fun and misery as well!

My first marriage was happy. I liked him very much – he was more like an older brother. He died suddenly, it was a heart attack. Then I met my second husband. I used to go out for a drink and he used to go in that pub occasionally. We got friendly and we did sleep together before we got married and it was much better, definitely, quite normal! He was very experienced and had had lots of women. We were very happy, it was different altogether from my first, that was quite happy in my mind but I had the happier one when I had a normal sexual relationship.

I'd had twelve years with this other man and suddenly I realised, 'Oh this is what I've been missing'. I've been quite a physical person. Of course lots of women put up with that situation all their married lives, nowadays girls won't, that's why people break up so easily. He died ten years ago. It was very hard.

Florrie is the kind of woman who always seems to have a man around. She enjoys their company and is somehow the type of woman that men go for. At the end of our interview, her current man, a handsome man in his sixties, comes in shyly and shakes hands. He glances at Florrie, a look of pure adoration, and she smiles back at him. Florrie considers herself lucky to have had a second chance – if her first husband had lived, she would have stayed with him and would never have had a chance of a happy sexual life.

Mary

Forty-seven. A hysterectomy plunged her into early menopause with terrifying speed and led to severe depression.

I was still a virgin when I met my second husband. I first got married when I was twenty and I separated after thirteen months. My second husband was a widower. I met him a year after I separated. We got married two and a half years after we met. I took on his three children. I had twin girls, Sue is a twin but we lost the other baby when she was nine months old. It's been very hard emotionally.

When I married my first husband, I had no experience of sex at all and it wasn't good, it was a disaster, an absolute disaster. He had no experience, so I'm all for the younger generation trying things out before marriage. I don't say to my daughter you mustn't do it, I just say if you are going to do it, make sure you are protected. I don't agree with sleeping around, like if you know some-one two weeks and you sleep with them. But if you are in a long-term relationship, after what happened to me, then I think it's fine. I wouldn't like her to go through all that.

Sex was one of the causes of our divorce. My mum told

me nothing about sex at all. This sounds really stupid to say now, but I really believed when I put that ring on my finger that everything was just going to fall into place! I must have thought that by magic . . . I don't know what I thought really.

Sex was a shock because I knew nothing at all about it. I couldn't respond to my husband at all. There's got to be a physical attraction there first and then you've got to be compatible. I was physically attracted to my first husband, very much so. We first went out together when I was about fourteen, but we were both too shy. We started going out again when I was fifteen, but we didn't sleep together – my mother had told me it was wrong and you didn't do it, totally the wrong upbringing.

You take it on board, you don't get over anything, you never have a clean slate again, as much as you would like to. I never managed to have sex with my husband, and we never went away on passionate weekends or anything like that. We came close to having sex in the lounge, we'd cuddle, but I was really repressed in that sense. It does affect your whole life, my mother had brought me up that way, that's why I was conscious that I wanted to be very different with Sue. Because I don't want to do anything she will have to carry with her all her life, I want to be a better mother than that.

There was no idea at all that sex could be fun, there weren't even really many books about. I was in love with my husband but it didn't work. Looking back I was very shy, fear as well and pain. I'm sure the difficulties I had with my first husband are what lots of women went through in the past. There again you see I thought I was on my own, I felt very isolated. There was no one I could talk to, I thought I was the only person it had ever happened to.

My mum was quite shocked when she realised that basically nothing was happening – everybody was shocked. It just hurt so much, I would freeze up. And he was worried about hurting me because it was so painful. Before we got married, you'd get to a point and then you'd stop. I met another fella then and I wondered if he took me away for the weekend, he could put it all right! But I didn't go. Where did we go from there? He didn't know what to do, it was tragic really.

I decided to leave because I thought it was going nowhere. If someone had talked to us, if we'd got counselling it might have helped. We would have had our twenty-fifth wedding anniversary last year. I'm sure there are women around now who got married when I did and who are suffering like I was. I often wonder about that, whether they are having affairs or completely finished with sex.

It seemed such a big thing, I went to marriage guidance. The counsellor conducted the whole interview with his flies undone! I don't know whether he was doing it on purpose, at one point he did leave the room and when he came back his zip was done up but I didn't know if it was some sort of test that I was supposed to comment on! I thought 'This is weird!'

Nobody really tells you what's what. Let's face it there's only a few basic points and everybody is always elaborating on them. Good sex is a combination of lots of things, it's not just where you put what. And basically tiredness, when you don't feel like it you think 'Is it worth it?'

I have had a quite a happy sex life with my second husband, but we have had so much to deal with. We had to get my divorce out of the way and I brought a lot of sexual problems to the marriage. Losing the baby was a big shock that took us a long time to get over. She had a bad heart and she had an operation but didn't survive. And then there were all the problems with his children. Then we had a good period and then he was made redundant, he went into business for himself and then he was ripped off there. We have both had illness, so we're just emerging again.

With my second husband, when we first got married, he worked four nights or five if he could get the overtime, so he was home in the afternoon, so sex was nice. When the babies were born we had all day when he woke up. You do get used to it, it's better not having to wait until night anyway, when you're tired, so it worked quite well.

When the baby died, the only reason I bothered with sex at all is because I wanted another baby, that was quite plain to him, that was grief. That gradually changed, it all came back all right!

When his business started to go wrong, he started having problems sexually and then I hurt my back. It's difficult to put your finger on what goes wrong when, it's a gradual thing, you don't always notice straight away. We have sex a lot less often but that is probably my fault, I don't feel like it so much and I feel that I don't need it. But I'm glad it's still in my life, I would hate to think that that was it, it is never going to happen again.

I've got a friend like that. She is only fifty-one and she is one of these people who said, 'Well I'm fifty now, so I should be feeling like this and I should be slowing down and it's about time I stopped having sex and feeling old and doing things that fifty year olds do.' I'm not like that, I don't believe that, I think you should do exactly what you want to do. Having a lot less sex is a problem from my husband's point of view. Men see it as you not fancying them. Maybe I don't fancy him so much but I'm not fancying anybody else either. It's just how I feel.

The difference between me and my daughter is that, even if I found it difficult to talk to my children about sex, I have talked to them both, it seemed really important. They would listen to what I said but they wouldn't actually respond. I don't now whether they were embarrassed or whether they thought 'Oh, here she goes again',

I don't know! I always made a point of talking to them about sex and not shutting them out from it, so it has always been quite open. There were lots of things I couldn't talk about but basically we do talk. And there is a big difference in the way my daughter is about sex to how I was.

My husband is a man's man. I suppose we must be quite tolerant because we have stayed together through all the problems. We just had each other but it is a miracle that we did survive. I've heard horror stories of people just walking out. We are very close emotionally although there are times when it gets too much. We do have a strong marriage, that is very lucky.

We've had a good physical relationship that has worked. I feel very affectionate towards him. We both look out for each other, although we have our ups and downs, when it comes down to it, we look after each other. Out of the two of us, if anyone was going to stray, it would be me. He's not that sort, but I have been tempted. I don't think looks count, I always look further down or rather, deeper! When you get to know someone, that's what counts, what's underneath. My husband isn't romantic, if he brings you a bunch of flowers they're not wrapped!

We've never been on our own as a couple. I had a four-day honeymoon and then came straight back to being a stepmother. We never had time to adjust, and I think you need time to build a relationship. That's the one thing I envy, if I envy anything about young people today. That's why I'd like to see both my children have a marriage first and then have children, because you have to build a foundation. We had to build that while looking after stepchildren and having our own children.

When Mary talked about her first marriage, she glossed over the difficulties to start with and just said they broke up. But there was a moment, a sort of tear in the atmosphere, when I felt something else was going on. Much later on in the interview she told me that she had still been a virgin when she married her second husband in the sixties. Her mother telling her that sex was not something to be enjoyed, but to feel guilty about, plus the automatic cut-off point with her fiancé when they felt they were 'going too far' during their courtship, made the likelihood of a good sexual relationship slim. I was fascinated that Mary thought of all those other women who had got married at the same time as her, and maybe had the same negative experience, at a time when everyone was supposed to be enjoying sex. The running theme throughout her life, through all the terrible years of depression at menopause and the tragic death of her baby daughter was that she felt she was on her own, despite the support from her second husband.

Maud

Seventy-eight. She is widow with three grown-up children. One of her daughters is also widowed. She has eight grandchildren.

I know one couple where when the wife had the menopause she said, 'That's it, no more sex with my husband' and I just couldn't understand that, she was rather that sort of person. I don't think she ever enjoyed sex and she was rather prudish and pleased to have an excuse to get rid of it. I never looked at menopause or periods as anything to do with children. I owe all that to Marie Stopes – she makes a big point of pleasure, and her book was called *Married Love*. I remember reading it and thinking it's not going to be one sided as I had thought!

With my parents, we didn't really talk about that sort of thing at all. I learnt about it from my schoolfriends and quite late actually, I was about seventeen before I knew the full story. My mother was very repressed. One day we met suddenly a mutual friend, who was very close to the family, who was very pregnant and who I knew wasn't married and it gave me a physical shock. She was coming out of a

cinema, she didn't see us but we saw her. It shocked me
so much that I could hardly see the film and I cried. In the
evening, my mother came to me and said, 'Aren't men
terrible?' That was enough to put me off anything for ever
afterwards! It was that sort of relationship.

I'll tell you how we had a good physical relationship.
Largely, it is because I read Marie Stopes' book before I
got married and that gave me the impression that it was
going to be a very enjoyable experience and that it was
going to be for both sides and that changed my attitude. I
don't think I would have got that idea from my mother.

My husband died in 1980 of a long illness, he was ill
really for almost ten years before he died. That didn't stop
us doing a tremendous lot of things. He retired at sixty
and he was quite a bit older than me – about eight years
older. We went and lived in Malta immediately after he
was retired, thinking that that would be a good idea. But
in actual fact it wasn't, the climate didn't really appeal to
him and I was homesick. Although my daughter was
married, she had a slightly shaky marriage I thought and
the two boys were not married at all. I kept on getting on
planes like buses, going backwards and forwards and
eventually we came home after four years. The years of
retirement were the happiest years of our marriage really.
I was very lucky, I look back on a very happy marriage, it
lasted forty-three years altogether.

I regarded menopause as a sort of freedom. My husband
and I were still having sex, and we had a very good sex life. I
think we were compatible, we were very much in love
almost to the very end of his life. And I think the last eleven
years after he retired we were closer than we had ever been.
He was ill a lot of that time so it was a different relationship,
much more of a caring one on my part. Unfortunately he
developed diabetes towards the end of his life, in the last
three or four years, which rendered him impotent.

We knew all about sex when we got married, but

neither of us were experienced. We had had a great deal of what is now called heavy petting, but we hadn't actually . . . I was a virgin but as I was rather scared of this, I got a doctor to cope with it, I'd rather he did it, so it was done with an instrument and that was that.

My husband was a very affectionate man, he wasn't thank goodness, what I call a macho man, I've never been attracted to any of that kind. Also we both had quite stable families, that has a great influence on people. They imagine that's what they've jolly well got to do for the rest of their lives.

There are two occasions in my married life that I think were important. One was right at the beginning, a few months after we were married, when suddenly I wanted to do something or other and he didn't want me to do it. So I said I would and he put his hands on my arms and tried to stop me physically. I said, 'That's it, I'll match you mentally in anything, but if you use force, never, never again will I have anything to do with you.' I walked out of the house at ten o'clock at night and it was December and I had a little parcel under my arm and I went off to the local pub and said I wanted a room.

It lasted about two days, then I couldn't bear it anymore and I went to the cinema and I suddenly heard his car with a special horn coming to meet me outside. Women have to be fairly strong. I'm absolutely not victim material, my mother probably was and I was always very determined not to be like her.

The other time was during the worst part of our marriage when he became very very involved in his business. I would have said at that time, that he was almost wedded to his business and I did what is known as a Shirley Valentine – do you know what I mean by that? I got really fed up, particularly as both my sons were in the business. I used to drive them all to the office and when they came home, it was business all the time.

I got so fed up that I went off to Tenerife by myself, which was extremely frightening but it made such a difference, our relationship immediately became right again straight away. I thought this was really important. It was in about 1966 when I was fifty. I told him I was going and he thought, and I think I encouraged it, that I was going out to an old boyfriend of mine who lived somewhere near there.

My brief escapade in Tenerife lasted about two months. I was absolutely terrified, going off on my own. What is more at the airport I had to get in this taxi and everything was dark and suddenly I remembered these awful stories about taxi drivers raping their customers. We went miles and miles and miles. I didn't know what the currency was like, so I thought I had better have a look at it. So I asked him, stupidly, to turn the light on and then I realised what I was doing, turning money out with him looking at it!

We finally arrived, it was Mardi Gras and a door was opened to me at this little hotel by somebody dressed up as the devil, it was absolutely appalling! Everybody was in fancy dress and I didn't know what to do. I went and sat at a table by myself and it was very frightening. But luckily next morning the sun came out and I went to the swimming pool and lay in the sun and it was all worthwhile.

He let me go and it was really quite cruel. Even one of my sons said, 'Do you mean to say that he is not even going to see you off?' It was the time that he was so wedded to his business, things were getting very exciting there and he was scared of his partner. I just thought 'That's it, I'm not going to have this sort of thing, I'm going to have some notice taken of me.'

On the way back, I decided for psychological reasons that I would delay coming back, so I got off the plane in the south of France where I had some friends. I did write at the last minute and said I'm not coming back on that day, I'm going to see so and so. Finally I arrived back about two weeks later than I should have and he was quite a different person. He met me at the airport and I didn't ever have any more trouble over the business!

It sounds awful doesn't it! I phoned and he wrote to me while I was away; it didn't disturb the essential relationship, it just showed him. One of my sons told me my husband was very distressed after I had gone. He was a proud man too, that was part of the reason that he didn't come and see me off, he wanted to show me that he didn't mind, go on then if you must.

I don't think I did it in a punishing way, I wanted to shock him more than anything else. It wasn't that it disturbed any big sexual thing, or anything of that kind, it was just that I didn't like the atmosphere and I wanted it changed. I didn't stray in Tenerife, there were one or two, men were interested by a woman on her own out there, so I had quite a lot of attention, which was nice.

The physical relationship with my husband improved a great deal over the years. We weren't frightfully inventive, as it seems everybody is nowadays, but it was very good and satisfying.

Of course when he had diabetes he became impotent, and that distressed him. He went to the doctor and said he was more worried about me than himself. The doctor told him there was very little that could be done. That took care of the last two years of our married life. Up to then we had been sleeping together regularly. I suppose it was more infrequent towards the end than it would have been earlier but we were still having sex.

He was upset at not being able to have sex but at a certain level, which may sound strange, after all I have said, he was an insensitive man. His emotions didn't go far, he was not very caring about other people. Perhaps it's just that female imagination and emotion goes just that bit deeper and you are always worrying about someone else. So once he had made me understand that he still loved me, but nothing more could happen, I think he probably just dismissed it, we were very affectionate physically.

Sex gets better with age and you know one another better. When he was ill, we still slept together, we kept our double bed, it was very affectionate. When he died I was holding his hand.

Maud stresses that she is not victim material and I can't help contrasting her experience of sex with Alice's, the walking disaster area. So what makes a woman like Maud take control and do a Shirley Valentine? Talking with her, it's clear that she has a very strong sense of self, who she is and what she is worth. That strong self-image is attractive to a different sort of man than the 'wasters' that Alice goes for. Like many other women of all ages I talked to, Maud had a repressive mother who was unable to talk to her about sex. Yet she managed to overcome that aspect of her background – the sexual happiness coming from the confidence and strong self-image, with a good dose of information, in this case, from Marie Stopes. Maud expected to have a good sex life and she did.

Dot

Seventy. She is married for the second time and has one daughter.

I was damaged goods already at twenty-four. It was very hard because all relationships were pretty tough. I had a very bad upbringing with a father who was the mayor of the local town. He abused me, so I was totally caught up in guilt. His abuse was not total abuse, in so far as I remember – although one never knows if there isn't something blanked out – but there was sufficient petting and playing with me and doing things to me that I knew were not right, and no one to talk to at all because I was sent away to boarding school at the age of eight. What was the point in telling anybody anyway? He was supposed to be the great, good man and he wasn't.

I fell in love at fourteen. He was the most divine creature who lived with us and he was on such a pedestal I thought he was really, really, really going to be my salvation. Nobody was told about this, but he was like a beacon of light from fourteen to eighteen. I thrived on this passion and he played up to me and one day we would marry. He was at least nine years older than me, lived in the house, nothing ever happened, it was just utterly idealistic which was exactly how I wanted it. Then just after my eighteenth birthday, he met somebody and married her within a week. I was away at boarding school and when my brother rang me with bad news, it was war time so I thought at first he had died.

I then had a lot of relationships in between him and my first marriage because I'd been through so much. Many relationships, but I knew nothing at all about sex! When I look back on it I remember seeing a man's penis for the first time when I was nineteen on a date with him in a hotel room, where we did not actually go the whole hog. I just didn't know what to look at, I thought what is this awful thing! It was incredible and I don't know how I came through to nineteen – mind you it was an erect penis, whereas I'd probably seen little bits before. We were so ignorant! I'd messed about, but not to that extent, to really know anything about men at all. No one had told me about sex, no way.

My first husband I met at university and he was beautiful to look at, absolutely divine and he had something very closed about him. Looking back now I should have known! I just set my cap for him, I thought this was going to be it. There were several others around and one of them would have been simply splendid, my mother's choice for me, but I thought he was much too good, and I was very much a rebel. I looked at all the wrong men, which my mother used to call picking up lame ducks, but really I was very innocent. I lost my virginity to a doctor, which was quite a good way to do it. I was about twenty. Nothing particularly nice happened, it wasn't a particularly interesting experience.

I fell for my husband in a rather calculated way, by this time I was beginning to play the part of being in love. I certainly knew that I wanted to marry this man, partly because I never felt that my self-image was much good, and therefore I felt it would make rather nice children to have a rather good-looking husband! That could be one reason. He was a Roman Catholic and totally against my parents' wishes. We ran away to London and then my brother caught up with us, so we were forced to get married, there was nothing for it, but I hadn't actually slept with him.

I know we may have got near to each other and played about a bit, but it seemed he was rather cold. But I thought that doesn't matter because I'm not that good at this game anyway, a complete failure, so it won't really matter if he is not too fast. I knew on the morning of the wedding that I shouldn't be going through with it. If I hadn't got married it would have been impossible for the whole family, nobody could have coped with me. I knew it was wrong, I felt terrified, I remember shaking all the way to the church, thinking 'I know this isn't right', just having to go on with it, because it just had to happen.

It was a dreadful mistake! On the honeymoon night he asked me to go out into the garden and get some birch twigs and I had to beat him. I was married then and caught in a trap. I couldn't tell anybody because I had been forced into it and there I was married to a man who was a psychopath.

He had these sexual deviations. It was a life of hell, I was terrified of him, he was violent if he didn't get his way. Sexually he had to be satisfied and it was gross and I couldn't really believe that this could happen. My doctor, who was such a gem of a man, said don't have a child by him. I talked to him and he said you must break this up but I didn't dare. I was too frightened of everybody – my father, my mother and my family. I was only twenty-four and immature. So we had a child within eighteen months, but even then I was already looking at other people. I remember having an affair in London – he was dishy. My husband was looking at other, more beautiful, people. I knew by that time I was a disaster as far as he was concerned, what he wanted was beauty.

It was a disaster all round. He wouldn't work, so I had to earn the living which supported us, even when I was carrying the baby. I had the baby; second-hand clothes, second-hand nappies even. I cannot see how I went through eleven years of it. But I did. In the end I only got away by meeting somebody who gave me the incentive. There were two or three instances where people would see me in a state and ask what the matter was. When I had affairs, it wasn't the particular man, it was me wanting the love, for God's sake somebody show me some compassion, genuine interest. Finally I ran away. I came to the point at which I could take the step but I was very, very frightened.

It was hair raising because I really didn't think I would survive, I thought he would kill me. I had had a domiciliary visit from a psychiatrist who said he must have help. I shall never forget, on the way downstairs, my husband looked at me and muttered, 'You wait until he's gone'. I was really frightened, the incidents were too awful to describe there were so many of them.

I wasn't allowed a divorce, my family only agreed to a separation, I was still under the family influence. I had no choice because they began to get wind that my life hadn't been pure and my husband said he thought I had been having an affair. My first husband looked too nice, I couldn't really tell them the truth, it was almost beyond their understanding and he could put on the most beautiful display and be utterly charming. So I was in a no-win situation. When they realised he would fight, they said I could only have a separation, it could not be brought into the courts, although I was willing to go through with the case. So I just let it be.

So for a long time we just had a separation and I had relationships. One in particular, with Christopher, was very pleasant – I'd known him when I was eighteen, and he was the one we went to when I ran away with my husband. Years later I got in touch with him and we immediately decided to live together, and we did so for two years, and then he had a heart attack and died. It was very sad.

Christopher had an accountant called Richard, and he said 'I only have one friend I want you to meet, my accountant'. So I knew Richard from earlier when he and his wife came to Christopher's flat. So my second marriage was almost arranged in the sense that I knew Richard, he was safe, he was lovely. His wife was killed in a car crash. I propped him up, as he had propped me up when Christopher died. I saw him through it and then we married. It's a long and complicated story!

If I had slept with my first husband before marriage, I would have known about him at once. If I had done what I had with other men even, it irritates me more than anything else that I had been so absurd. I wouldn't have married him at all, no way. So I didn't actually sleep with the person I ended up with first. I would always encourage anyone who is getting married to spend time with their partner. I'm so pleased there is a safe way of doing it now, and that people are allowed to morally. It's appalling, sex is not something you can work at, if it is really wrong. With his problems, there was absolutely no way that I should have gone on in that situation.

My second marriage has not been easy at all in the sexual sense. We have not got those great demands for each other and I thank God for it, because otherwise it would have been difficult.

I have never had a really good sexual relationship, never. Only if I didn't have them! That sounds stupid, but I do remember one man whose little finger I touched in a taxi and I felt like jelly and I realised then that was what sex was all about. I only needed to touch his little finger! We never ever went any further and he went off to Africa and asked me to go out and join him and I didn't dare, I was too frightened.

Richard and I didn't waste time, we married within sixteen months of his wife's death. We had both been through such a lot and he was still having nightmares. In the twenty-five years I could not count how many men I had before Richard. When he decided he was interested in me, because I waited quite some time, I said to him, 'But you don't know me', and he said, 'But I don't care. If I choose my wife, I choose her forever', and there was something in the way he said it. From then on I've had twenty-five years of not having anything intimate with any other man and I feel rather proud of it. It was partly because of his outlook, there was no way I could two time him, I just never felt the same. He's the right person in many ways.

Sexuality is about lots of other things – the way you relate to other people, how affectionate you are. There is a lot of warmth in so many relationships that I have enjoyed and still enjoy. Sex is reduced to penetration these days and it's got to be well handled and it often isn't. The word foreplay now is all over the place, and thank God for that, but we didn't know what it was and nor did men. So we often started off with something that felt so ghastly that it rather put you off anyway.

Sexuality is not really about sex. I know what an

orgasm is and I can masturbate and I can get halfway there. I would adore, before I die, to have the wonder of the experience of the terrific thing! But I still don't think it's as terrific as that, because I believe that I have come to something even better in certain types of meditation. I believe I know what is beyond it. That's as far as I can go, I think one gets as far as one can at this game.

The abuse Dot suffered at the hands of her father, that she had to keep secret for so many years, reinforced her feelings of low self-worth. She then picked a man who turned out to be a psychopath for her first husband and was bound to him, literally, by the social prejudices of her family. Despite her many sexual liaisons, she has never managed to have an orgasm, though her longing has not disappeared, which she deals with in a humorous way. It's hardly surprising that she was on tranquillisers for so many years nor that she had such a desperately difficult menopause. Yet Dot says herself that menopause has allowed her finally to come to terms with her life.

Chapter Three

Fidelity

If you read the papers or watch television you could easily come to the conclusion that the only faithful couple in history were Adam and Eve, and you know what happened to them. Fidelity is a non-starter in terms of the sexy stories that feed the media, apart from the odd golden wedding couple who are used as icons to make the rest of us feel inadequate and guilty. They've generally not spent a night apart since their wedding day, where most of us would give anything to have the odd night off. Yet in real life, infidelity is clearly a major cause of marriage break-up; either because one partner has gone off with someone else, or had an affair in order to bring dissatisfaction within the marriage out into the open.

This chapter looks at the whole question of fidelity. This was a difficult topic, and I had to recognise that this chapter was the most likely to produce evasive answers. Would women be willing to say they had wanted or indeed had affairs? How important was fidelity in a long-term relationship, was it indeed possible? What happened when partners were unfaithful, did they automatically leave? Would there be differences in the generations? And what about people who weren't married, did they consider themselves to be bound by the same rules? Was flirting an important safety valve in long-term marriages and how did partners work out their problems? I was surprised again by the honesty and frankness of the responses.

Until death us do part is still true for the older generation of women I interviewed. When they married, most of them knew nothing about sex and would not have entertained the idea of an affair for one moment. Once married, they had no expectations about sex or sexual fulfillment for themselves, regarding it more as a duty to perform to fulfil the man's needs. The idea of a woman getting pleasure from sex was not discussed: a woman found happiness in the efficient maintenance of the home and through her family and children. The social codes of the day were rigidly enforced, and divorce was shameful. Social pressures were immensely strong, not just from the establishment, but from the neighbourhood. One woman reported her family's obssession with the neighbours; their views and prejudices were paramount, nothing must be done to upset them, cause comment or lose the good name of the family. Anything that might hint at immorality or pregnancy before marriage, such as a teenager coming home late on her own, was frowned upon. The aura of respectability must be maintained.

Class, of course, made a difference. One middle-class woman had an open marriage with her husband and they both had affairs. A woman before her time, she moved in artistic circles and believed that sexual pleasure was as important for herself as for her husband. Even more shockingly for the time, she didn't really believe in marriage at all, but got married because of the war. She eventually divorced her husband for cruelty many years later, when he became an alcoholic. For her, fidelity was a nonsense, an impossible standard, but she was an exception among the women I spoke to.

Most women in their fifties and sixties will have faced advances from men, either in the work place or in social situations. The pattern has changed as women have become more liberated, some men assuming that women are available for sex. Jobs which involve travel and meeting a lot of people provide opportunities and excuses.

Coping with the grope was embarrassing for them, because it changed the balance of power at work. Many women were surprised when advances were made to them; one said that she thought men had a sexual agenda all the time, while women only thought of sex intermittently.

Men and women have different agendas when flirting. Men are on the pull, looking for any strays they can single out from the herd. Women are just jousting and reported anxiety when they were taken seriously (by being rung up the following day, for example) out of the context of the party.

The work situation provides the other rich vein of flirtation material. One woman reported living a fantasy flirtation with a work colleague because she was having sexual problems with her husband. When I asked her if she would be prepared to put fantasy into action she looked horrified, the whole point of the fantasy flirtation was that it remained only in the realm of the imagination.

Trust was the key to strong relationships. The ability to keep a husband on a long, loose leash paradoxically seemed to remove a need to stray. It boiled down to trust and communication – if all was happy at home, there was no need to look elsewhere. But when trust disappeared, it spelt death for the relationship. One woman put a detective on her husband's tail and discovered he had a baby with someone else.

Many of the women felt that my generation didn't work hard enough at relationships, that we went off with the first temptation that came along and didn't stick with problems and try and work them out. But women of my generation find it difficult to imagine sleeping with the same partner for a lifetime. We have been brought up to expect more from relationships: sexual pleasure, companionship, equality, and to maintain these with the same person for forty years seems to be a Herculean task. Women in the past seemed to try harder or perhaps they simply put everyone else before themselves, their own needs came a poor fifth to the demands of the rest of the family. Yet if a relationship is to work, it must necessarily involve putting the other partner's needs first – of course this should be reciprocal.

The shelves of bookshops are groaning under the weight of the 'me first' philosophy of life, but if a 'me first' meets another 'me first', how are they ever going to make a satisfactory relationship? Being brought up in the consumer age makes fidelity in marriage and long-term relationships unfashionable. If you live in a society which grazes rather than sits down to meals, where if you get tired of your car, you simply buy another one, how can you resist trading in your partner for a new model, when the first scratches on the paintwork appear?

Brenda

Fifty-four. She smiles with delight when talking about her husband. There is a strong sexual bond between them.

Good sex brings stimulation and closeness. I haven't strayed and I don't know whether he has – I would say he hasn't, but you never ever really know. I've been tempted. I'm a little bit naïve to think that anyone would fancy me and I probably give off the impression that I'm happily married. But I worked for a sales company and I had a rep taking me round – I must have been in my forties. He brought me home from this conference and I must have dozed off in the car and I found that he stopped the car and I thought we were home. He put his hand on my hand bent over and kissed me! I thought, 'Oh my God, what do I do now?' and I said to him, 'You're half my age, you can't do this, it's not right'. Then he said he would like to take me out. I was only concerned that he was so much younger. It was only when I was speaking to a close friend of mine and she said, 'Gosh did that boost your ego?' and I'd missed it [*she laughs*] but it wouldn't cross my mind to do anything about it. It would rock my boat.

I don't know how I would feel if my husband did anything, because you can say, 'Oh yes, our love is very strong', lots of brownie points, but how strong is it if that happens? He'd have to do something first . . . We must be very boring.

I don't envy my younger daughter and her experience, and that makes me sound really boring, doesn't it! Perhaps if I could go off and come back and for everything to be exactly the same, then I suppose yes, I might, but I would want to know a lot about them. But I feel that it would just spoil everything.

Brenda's strong sexual partnership with her husband has meant that she has not been tempted to look elsewhere. She gives off such clear signals of being happy in herself, I would be surprised if she hadn't had many more advances that she simply hasn't noticed. She thinks of herself as boring because she is happily married – that may be a result of the pernicious influence of the media and particularly lipstick journalism in some women's magazines with their continual repetition of performance hit parades and articles explaining fifteen ways to the essential orgasm. Masquerading as information, in fact it is designed to keep women worried about their sexuality and in a constant state of self-doubt and worthlessness.

Marjorie

Seventy-six. She is divorced but she had an open marriage which she very much enjoyed.

I enjoyed my sexual life with my husband – it was only the sexual life that in the end kept me with him, because the marriage finally tapered off. There was no change in the sex. Before you get married, sexual compatibility is probably chance, that's why I would never get married until I had slept with somebody. I mean, damn it, if I buy a pair of gloves, I'm allowed to try them for size. I think it's a big mistake not to, a very grave error.

You don't have to get bored, even in a long marriage, if you know what you're doing and how to do it. Even after thirty years. I don't call having affairs straying, it's essential that you have good definitions. When we got married, it was quite understood or it was quite implicit. I told him I didn't give a damn what he did, I knew he loved me and I loved him, all I said was, that if he wanted to have a bit on the side, or whatever the expression was in those days, so far as I was concerned there were only three provisos. That he didn't get anything that neither of us wanted, that he didn't spend too much time away and that he didn't spend any money that we couldn't afford. And I think that was fair enough. I felt that what was good for the gander was good for the goose.

I had one or two affairs, why not, if I wanted to, if the going was possible? But affairs are an awful lot of trouble – if you don't want to rub anybody's nose in it. I don't think it matters to either person, as long as they don't think other people know about it, that's what's humiliating for a man and a bit of a triumph for a woman and that's why you kick him out. So you do your bad, if bad it is, by stealth.

I believe the popular term today is relationships, it's a word I can't stand, it sends me up the fucking wall! Some of them would last one night, two nights . . . you went somewhere and you liked somebody it took a long time, you met them one day and then something happened. Very hard to say what attracts me; must have a good sense of humour, must think very much as I do. There are some about, you'd be surprised! Must love animals too. I would never stay with anybody or live with anyone else. I never wanted to.

Marjorie's candour about relationships and affairs shows that some women of her generation were able to live in a completely modern way. This was a matter of education but also of class; working-class women were less independent financially and more dependent on the close-knit family and social group which exercised a restraining, moralistic influence. Middle-class artistic women like Marjorie, who were financially independent and mixed in artistic circles, had more liberal attitudes to sex and fidelty than many young women today.

Annie

Fifty-six. She is a single gay woman who was left after a long-term, live-in relationship ended in acrimony.

Fidelity is important to me. I have never ever cheated on anybody, mentally I might have done, but sexually never. I am by nature monogamous, a very unfashionable thing to say! Terrible, but I am, if I'm with somebody I'm with that person and that's where my thoughts go. I couldn't cheat because I wouldn't have wanted to hurt her.

I'm very insecure about practical things. When I lost my house and my relationship, I just felt as though my life had totally broken down. I tend to be a bit clingy in relationships, which is maybe why I don't want to get into another one because I don't want to cling like that again. I wouldn't want to live with anybody, because I know I can get stuck with a bad relationship – our relationship was not good but I clung on to it because of the house and the way of life.

Annie stressed that her long-term relationship had been similar to any heterosexual relationship: cats, a shared mortgage, rows about the decorations. But when the relationship broke up, through her partner's infidelity, Annie felt doubly lost because she was not 'out' as a gay woman and could not talk about the loss she felt to anybody.

Katherine

Fifty-three. She has been married all her adult life to the same man. There are difficulties in their sexual relationship, which she is coming round to tackling.

I have been tempted to stray several times. It's very strange, because if I did stray I'm sure I would be terribly upset about it. I would feel that I had betrayed something and I think about how I would feel if he did the same to me.

The temptation is to think, if he doesn't know how can it hurt, but suppose I did stray and then it became serious, I would really be hurting him and I don't want to take that risk. I have a colleague at work who I fancy desperately, but I know that if it came to the moment, I would be absolutely terrified.

As far as I know, we have both been faithful to each other. My husband is the sort of old-fashioned chap who thinks that it's a betrayal of somebody and everything is focused on the one person, which is a bit of a burden at times. Perhaps a little bit of fun might have opened his eyes a bit. I have been seriously tempted a couple of times with different people. The situation and circumstances were ideal but the panic button is pressed and I withdraw very quickly and make excuses.

Though I say that I'm much more secure in my body and my feelings about myself now, there's that deeply embarrassing thing about the fact that you've got to take your clothes off at some point, or bits of them at least! Hopefully in the heat of the moment that wouldn't matter.

I'm sure part of it is fancying, rather than doing anything about it. I had a couple of lovers before my husband, and it was always slightly disappointing after waiting. The fancying bit went on for quite a while, because in my day you didn't sleep with someone on your ninth date, never mind the first! Maybe that was the problem, you were expecting so much it was bound to be disappointing.

Katherine's rich fantasy life – dreaming about colleagues at work and fancying young men on the bus home – is her way of coping, at the moment, with an unhappy sexual relationship with a dearly loved husband. She indicates that menopause has been a turning point in acknowledging her dissatisfaction, and that if she is unable to resolve her problems with her husband she is closer to straying now than she ever has been.

Alice

Sixty. She has been married twice and is now living with her first husband again. Both husbands messed around with other women.

Fidelity has been very important to me. I expect it from other people and I want to be faithful myself because you make a contract, it's rather like working, there's a loyalty. I expect that from my partner. If I had discovered that they were cheating on me, I would have walked straight out of the door with no compunction because they would have reneged on our agreement. I can't forgive it because I would never do it myself, unless we'd broken down. I'd already decided to leave my second husband when I bumped into my first husband again.

A woman of strong principles, Alice has nevertheless put up with a lot from both her husbands. She even went to the length of engaging a detective to follow them and make sure they were being faithful to her. If you can be that suspicious of someone you live with, how could you possibly take up with them again more than twenty years later?

Rose

Eighty-four, now widowed. She married for better or worse — her husband suffered many years of illness.

He never used to make love at all much. As a young man he contracted TB. I was never tempted to stray, ooh, gosh no! You were brought up to think it was a terrible thing to do, that kind of thing. To me, it would like be on my mind the rest of my life, to do something like that. So I just accepted the situation.

People did have affairs secretly, I'm sure they did, but it all had to be done very secretly. When I worked at the water board, there were porters there and I know one or two women used to lark about and they would chase them, all that kind of thing. I was always tall with blonde hair and I was cleaning up one day and one of the men there, in his late twenties, I remember him coming up and saying 'You're just the girl I'd like', and he put his arm round me. I was shy, I didn't know what to do. And when I got home I thought, 'Ooh he'd taken notice of me', which my husband didn't take! It gave me a little boost!

Rose spoke fondly of her husband and described her marriage as being happy. If she resented anything, it wasn't so much a lack of sex with her husband as the fact that he never took much notice of her. Rose describes herself as painfully shy, so flirtation was never an option for her. But other men found her attractive and flirted with her, and although she had no idea what to do, it lifted her spirits. Her face lit up with pleasure when she was recounting what happened at the water board more than fifty years ago. It highlighted the waste of affection and love in so many women of her generation whose husbands just never thought to compliment them.

Madeleine

Seventy-three. She has the happiest marriage of the whole group. Her face lights up when she talks about him, and when he drives me to the station later, he says he is so happy with her that he really does not want to die yet.

Lots of people can't imagine sleeping with the same person all that time. Why it has lasted I don't know, because if you'd asked me that when I was twenty, I'd have said you must get bored with the same person and there aren't any new tricks. But if you always have this wonderful experience you don't want to change. People who go off and try and find someone else are really trying to find something even better than they have got.

I would expect sexual expectations to decline after the first year or two of ecstasy [*she laughs*]. I suppose then it's getting off to work and getting the children off and all that, but by no means did it stop, we were always very happy to be together.

I haven't been tempted to stray, well just once, quite seriously, and looking back I don't know why really. It was just the exotic south of France and a millionnaire you know, that was the one time that I was tossing it up. The thought of twenty-five years with one man – what was on the other side of the fence? But no, what it comes back to, is could I hurt him that much and I couldn't, so it didn't come to anything. It wasn't worth the upset it would have caused and he could have been devastated, and now looking back I made the right decision.

Fidelity is important, you have to have a pact. I've always said if you find you want to go and have this experience by all means go and do it. I would prefer not with anybody I know. If you feel there is something inadequate in our relationship, go and come back and I don't really wish to know about it. And because he has had me allowing him permission, I don't think he's needed to stray. It's very strange, I always feel if you hold them down with reins, they want to break away. I have a very basic confidence in the relationship – we are very confident with each other.

Christopher has always said that as soon as he met me that was it, I was the one for him. We saw each other from a distance and I wasn't interested, I had another boy-friend at the time. We went to a dance and he asked me to dance and as soon as he put his arms round me that was it! It felt perfect and he felt it as well and it's the same now, if he puts an arm round me, it feels the same for both of us, so I've always known that he would come back, that he would be there.

I don't flirt much now, in a friendly way maybe. But when I was younger – Christopher is very very jealous, so he went through a rotten old time until he realised that he could trust me.

We fit very well, I think it was ordained, somebody up there said these two need each other! Looking around my friends, I know the way some of them talk about their partners behind their backs, they score points, bitterness, it's a war going on. They've missed the point and I stop them sometimes and say to them, think back to why you got married, what was the urge that made you want to be with that man and where is that now.

Our sexual problems [*painful intercourse since menopause*] haven't affected me so much, I've been disappointed that

Christopher has been deprived of this outlet in a way, but he never complains about it. He says it would be lovely if we could, but he wouldn't dream of hurting me or anything like that, so he's come to terms with it and it doesn't enter my head very much at all, I am so busy. It would be lovely, if this **HRT** worked wonders, it would be wonderful.

The confidence Madeleine and her husband feel in each other, that their bond is for life, has allowed them to imagine the other partner's infidelity and come to terms with the possibility in an adult way. Madeleine's policy of loose reins on her husband has clearly been a positive experience for them both – why go out for a hamburger when you have steak at home?

Mavis

Seventy-three. She married twice, happily the second time, and is now widowed. She is still sexually active.

Fidelity is very important. If you live with someone and you love them then you have to trust them, so if they're not faithful there is no point in going on. You can't have a complete relationship if you haven't got complete trust.

If you get on well and have a happy and satisfying sexual relationship, even after many years of marriage there's no need to look around. You've got to work at sexual compatibility, it's like everything else, you've got to work at it.

Mavis has recently finished an affair with a much younger man who was married. She felt that his marriage was his responsibility, not hers, and was happy to relinquish him when he wanted to go back to his wife.

Jenny

Fifty-four. Her marriage broke up at menopause, in part because her husband was having an affair with a neighbour. She is now divorced with three children, and is dating again after a long period of counselling.

I was never tempted to have affairs. Fidelty is very important to me. He went off with the lady five doors away. He said for a long time it wasn't a sexual affair and I believed him because he wasn't interested, he had totally lost interest in sex. I was very upset when we broke up, but it didn't put me off men altogether, not at all, I like men a lot.

I never felt that, because I had a good marriage for a long time. He was a nice man, a bit weak, I was a much stronger personality, much more dominant and I suppose I got fed up being the dominant one. I would have liked someone stronger really. I always liked him, we were always great friends so I never thought, 'Oh sod men, I never want to see another one as long as I live', not at all! I was very hurt though, very upset.

It took six months before I had another relationship! I didn't intend to at all. I went on holiday to Greece, it was a singles group and I met a man there. We were just friends in Greece but he wanted to see me when we came back to England and it developed from there.

The break-up with my husband didn't make me sexually nervous, not in the early days, if anything it has now, strangely enough. It didn't last, he wanted to get married, he was very keen. I wasn't though, I hadn't been on my own long enough. He said, 'Hurry up and decide, if you don't want me, I'm going to go and look for someone else!' I was still upset and in tears a lot of the time about my marriage breaking up. He was very intolerant about that and would say things like, 'For goodness sake that was six months ago'. Quite amazing! His wife had died six months previously and he had got over it just like that.

Since then, I've had a lot of men friends which has been very nice. I lacked confidence because of my mother. She always said they were very superior and we should be subservient to them, so I never ever had any men friends; I was frightened of them, they were a race apart. I've got a lot of nice friendships with men now – not sexual relationships – they ring me to ask me how I am and are quite protective. I had an affair a couple of years ago. I met a new man a lot older than me – he was sixty-five – but seemed very young with a lot of vitality. It came to a disastrous end because I have found that older men in their sixties are very keen to prove their sexual prowess.

I was really nuts about him, we got on very well and eventually went to bed together and he couldn't manage it, he was completely impotent and that really shook him terribly. He was a widower and it was the first relationship he had had since his wife had died. He said, 'I can't cope with my feelings and emotions and I shall never have another woman as long as I live'. That was awful, because I tried to talk about it and say these things do happen sometimes.

Now I've got a new man, we met through an ad in the paper. I met him once for a drink and he was all right. I gave him my phone number, thinking he would never ring but he did. I was amazed really and we've been out a lot since, it seems to be going OK. I'm spending my first weekend with him this week. I'm more confident with men, I know what I want and what I don't want.

I went out with a guy about a year ago for a few nights. He very much wanted a sexual relationship, but I didn't, he wasn't what I wanted. He was weak again, I could recognise this, he wasn't dominant, it was 'Yes dear, no dear anything you say dear, not if you don't want me to dear', deeply unsexy! It's a real turn off. He'd say, 'I can't bear to be parted from you, I want to spend every minute with you', and I was thinking 'Oh my God! Give me some space'. I ran off in the opposite direction.

I want someone positive and decisive and strong. I'm strong and I want someone who reflects that. I've got no respect for weak men. I had a very deprived childhood from an emotional point of view, I never had any love. I need someone strong and very loving, I know that. Men find it difficult to be both, though some of them are. I suppose it depends on their past as well, of course.

I don't like younger men, they don't appeal. I'm very aware of the aging process and very aware that my arms and legs are getting saggy, so I would feel sexually embarrassed with a younger man. I feel sexually more comfortable with a man about my own age or slightly older.

Dating isn't hard, I just get fed up with it, I get fed up getting to know them. It's fine if they're just going to be mates, you can go out for a drink and just have a laugh and a good time. But if it's a bit more serious, you do get fed up, is this going to work or is it another one that is going to hit the dust? I would like someone a bit more permanent. I'm not saying I want to get married. I like the idea of having a bit of space and seeing them at weekends, I wouldn't mind living with someone if I felt right about it.

I like the anticipation, like this weekend – will it go any further? I find it difficult to make the first move, it is something I have thought about. It's a difficult one, because you're always afraid of rejection if you make the first move. On the other hand, I've got to in this situation because he's let his feelings be known. We went out to dinner and he was holding my hand and gazing into my eyes and saying where do we go from here, he wanted to see lots more of me, but that if he got possessive I must tell him, if I wanted my own space. And he left it at that, wanting answers, so the next move has got to come from me. He did the first handholding, but I was ready for that. I felt a bit of a dickhead, as my daughter would say, sitting there in the restaurant with this man holding my hand and gazing into my eyes! It was something that had never happened to me before, it was really quite nice. Very new and very public and that was quite nice in itself, it was very reassuring.

I'm really floundering about the next move. We're going walking tomorrow, then he's cooking a meal, then we're going for a drink because he wants me to meet his friends. I am a bit concerned that I'm going back to his house to sleep, I'm not ready to sleep with him yet, but he's obviously aware of that. Age doesn't make any difference at all to knowing what the next right move is. Will he half hint or say he'd like to sleep with me or show me into another bedroom? If I'm honest, I'd quite like him to say that he would like to sleep with me, I don't just want to get shown into the spare room! It is very awkward when you're not communicating terribly well on an emotional level. I'm hoping that if we go walking that we can talk. See how it goes. It's great having someone fancy you, it does such a lot for your self-esteem!

Men have often told me that they fancy me, but I haven't fancied them, which has been a shame. I feel I'm on the brink of another relationship, but I'm nervous, a bit frightened that he doesn't feel the same. He is probably feeling all this as well. He's said he wanted to see lots of me, but I'm still frightened to say anything in the same vein. I'm frightened of rejection, of thinking this is wonderful, it's going really well, and then it doesn't and you're back to square one again.

But I don't really want to take it slowly either! I'd like to plunge in with both feet, have a really nice affair with him, but I'm very cautious and frightened that I shall end up with egg on my face. Men don't always tell the truth, they are very good at lying. I don't think they do it deliberately – they mean it at the time. This is why I'm being so cautious.

After a difficult divorce, Jenny is ready to strike out on her own again, but her low self-confidence makes it difficult for her to trust that when men say that she is wonderful, they really mean it. She has also been out with some lemons, which doesn't help in the self-confidence stakes. Nothing changes, this mature woman in her fifties is having the same doubts and worries about herself as her teenage daughter. Does he like me? Can I trust him? How far should we go?

Florrie

Eighty-four. She has had two marriages and now has a live-in boyfriend in his sixties. Her first marriage was not a sexual success although she describes it as happy. Her second marriage worked sexually.

During marriage I was never tempted to stray. I've not really had other relationships, I'm not the kind that people go for, a bit of a mouse. I've got someone living here – a man very nice, marvellous to me. He is my boyfriend I suppose, though we're a bit old for that word. He's younger than me, about sixty-seven. He probably would like sex but it doesn't bother me, I'm not that worried. But he's a nice man, we sleep together in the same bed, and it's nice to have someone around. He's very good, breakfast in bed every morning without fail! He does all the shopping and he can cook and garden.

We met in the park, walking the dog! Even when I was married we would pass the time of day. His wife died and my husband died and we were both a bit lonely and I suppose because I was a bit lonely, we got to talking more and mentioned that we had lost our partners. But he was the one who was keen, I didn't mind really. I've always had men friends around, always. I get on well with them, they talk about different, more interesting things. Some women are interesting, but in general I prefer men. Perhaps they like me because I am quiet! I let them talk, that might be the secret!

I haven't really got my feet on the ground, never have really. I was surprised and my daughter thought it was a hoot. He came round with a bottle of wine and a big box of chocolates and said he would like to go out with me. I told my daughter that I had a follower! She said 'Go for it mum, you go out with him'. She encouraged me no end, she loved the idea. Lots of people are lonely in life, I've not been alone for long.

I'm not really awfully interested in sex. I wouldn't seek it, I liked it when it happened, it was enjoyable. I like the companionship, I don't like being alone. I don't flirt, if they come to me, I'll talk to them, I'm not frightened of men but I have never sought their company.

Florrie has never sought men's company but has not been alone for long in her life. She clearly appeals to men. Her first marriage was not happy sexually but she was not tempted to stray, she just accepted that's how things were. She belongs to the generation that believes in getting on with things. Her explanation that her appeal lies in her listening to men and keeping quiet is said with a gleam in her eye, she certainly doesn't seem like the mouse type to me!

Mary

Forty-seven. An early hysterectomy plunged her into a terrible menopause which caused severe depression. She married twice, and was still a virgin when she married her second husband.

I'm not tempted to stray at all. I see men very differently now. They don't interest me, it's as though they all come out the same! I don't think much of men really, over the years there have been a lot of men I could have strayed with, put it like that. Even now I still rate a second glance, but I don't really care if they give me a second glance or not. Ten years ago, it was nice to think that someone found me attractive. Men used to fancy me at work, so if I'd wanted to stray, I could have done. But I didn't because of a deep-seated loyalty. It was also a sexual thing, because I wasn't on the pill I could have caught for a baby, or AIDS. Deep down I didn't want to be unfaithful. I'd say thank you, but no thank you. I don't like to hurt people's feelings and even when men used to hassle me, I found it difficult to say 'Will you go away and leave me alone!' I still find it hard now and I suppose this is a lack of assertiveness. Men are funny, they assume you must be available for them. It was difficult sometimes and caused all sorts of problems at work.

I get on well with men but I find that it's very difficult to just have men friends, they always tend to try and take it that bit further. I did have one I liked, I trusted him a lot. I could talk to him without it going any further or feeling that he would take advantage of the situation. Men would come on to me a lot and flirt with me. Sometimes I wanted to have some fun, my husband was working nights, I saw flirting as just a release for me, I could go out with my friends and have a laugh. Basically it was, I will flirt and that is it. There was nothing else.

There's been more than one I have been tempted by, but knowing deep down that I would never go and do anything. My family and children are very important to me and I would never do anything to hurt them. I know I'm attractive to men and it is nice in a way, but it can cause ructions. People think you're after their partner and the other women think it's you and not their husbands.

Mary seems to have a strange mixture of feelings about fidelity. Clearly attractive to men, with her blonde hair and slim figure, she likes to flirt with men but also despises them. She's the type of woman other women would perceive as a threat because she enjoys flirting. The importance of her home and family life and the stability they have brought her through many years of difficulty mean that she would be reluctant to jeopardise them for an affair with a man she at heart despised.

Maud

Seventy-eight. She was happily married for many years and is now widowed.

We worked sex out together, I don't think he'd had much experience before. The awful thing was that we were separated for three years during the war, two years after we were married – that was terrible. What was quite nice and perhaps rather significant, was that when he came home, I said to him, 'Now have you been faithful to me?' and sometimes he used to say 'Good gracious no, what in three years?' Other times, he used to say 'I've been faithful to you for every minute of the time'. And I used to say the same thing and neither of us knew whether it was true. It wasn't entirely true on my part. It was a difficult time, the war, you know.

Many people strayed during the war. I'm afraid that was fairly typical. At one point all the Americans arrived and I didn't really, properly stray then, but nearly all my friends did. It wasn't until later on in the war that I met a young Jewish officer and we had an affair. It was different, he was certainly quite experienced. The great thing that has always been true with me is that I'm only attracted to people intellectually, I'm hardly ever interested in anybody otherwise. They have to make themselves interesting to me before I start thinking in terms of falling in love or anything like that.

He was a very clever man, he had trained as a doctor

and got pushed into the army. I never had any other contact with him after my husband came home, but I had friends in London who were also doctors and I knew what he was doing. I did want to see him again, partly out of curiosity, to see what had happened to him. But I don't think I would have been interested in anything else.

Looking back I'm very glad I did have other experiences, it's more interesting and you are incomplete if a woman only has one man. I'm pretty sure that my husband had some experience when he was in India.

We both always said the same thing, either that I had been riotously unfaithful with every man I came across, or nothing at all. Neither of us ever knew. I accepted it, I thought it was best, I had something to hide too. I was not really tempted to stray afterwards. I remember someone once at a big business dance was paying me an awful lot of attention and I thought afterwards it would be rather nice if he were to take me out and I admit I rang him up, I think my husband was in the next room when I did it! But this man was wise enough not to do it! I don't think I would ever have slept with him, but I would have enjoyed his company.

I have a feeling that wives have been very jealous of me. I've been told that I've got a sort of fluffy, female outlook and they think that their husbands are attracted. It's happened several times although I don't think that I am very attractive to men. If I go to a party I wear rather flowing clothes.

It once caused terrible trouble, I discovered that a friend thought I was having something with her husband. I had absolutely no idea and it was absolutely untrue. I remember a party with a group of people, all laughing and talking. Her husband was in the group and I was holding the floor a bit. There were other men and women there. Next time they had a party – we were quite close as a foursome – they didn't invite us and I laughingly rang them up and said what have we done? It wasn't until the wife died, about fifteen years later, that someone said to me that she thought I was having a relationship with her husband!

When I was a lot younger I was quite pretty, the sort of prettiness that a lot of women would think would attract men although I don't think it did ever. Women are always afraid of other beautiful women. I looked at one or two of them with my husband too, the girls who worked in his office. I think men are attracted by the physical straight away, they take one look at a beautiful woman and wonder what she is like in bed. I've always felt that I never attracted men easily, but that all their wives were jealous, it was rather difficult. I used to rather emphasise the intellectual to counteract the other, but I was always vain enough to enjoy making myself attractive, out of self-respect. It's very easy to slip into slovenly habits, especially at my age, that's why I'm quite careful about it. I'm not good at flirting because I like the intellectual side and they don't go together. I'm not good at being coy and come hithering at all, that's what most people expect.

Maud was quite open about her infidelity during the war, and suggested that it was almost universally true among her peer group of respectable married women. They mostly went back to their husbands at the end of the war, and didn't ask too many questions of their husbands. Maud believes it did her marriage good; they both had more experience. Her attractiveness to men, and the hostility that she has experienced from other women, show how much women are taught to see their husbands as catches, to be clung on to and defended against all comers. All other attractive women then become a threat. It seems sad that a close friend would suspect her of infidelity but not feel able to discuss it with her. Maud is an interesting contrast with Madeleine's attitude, who felt so convinced by the rightness of her relationship, that she was prepared to let her husband stray, confident that he would eventually return.

Dot

Seventy. She married twice, the first time to a man she describes as a psychopath.

Fidelity to me is what Richard set me as a standard. It certainly didn't exist before, because all I craved for was being loved and I really thought that if people wanted my body they loved me, of all the naïve thoughts! It took so long to realise that it was nothing to do with that. The greatest friend I have is a man in Devon, a man who wanted me and who never had me and it's just a joy to go there. He knows that had he had me, we could never be the friends we are, at the level we are. I'm so pleased with that.

I love men and I like attractive men. I certainly have the same urges and I know when a person likes me. I know people I wouldn't dream of bedding, but on the other hand you know it is a little bit more than a kiss when it's a certain sort of kiss! Having a warm relationship and knowing that it is going no further doesn't matter at all as long as they also know that.

Dot's history of sexual infidelities and liaisons is clearly linked to the sexual abuse she suffered as a child, and the low self-worth that arose from that. Her compulsive need to be loved – while at the same time choosing unsuitable lovers, who could never provide what she craved because it has to come from within – has made her sexual history tortuous. She also talked about her inability to achieve orgasm, despite her numerous partners. Her relationship with her second husband has given her the calm and space to examine herself and come to terms with the horrors of the past. It is significant that menopause was the moment when she finally felt able to face herself.

Chapter Four

Men

'Pigs, selfish, lazy bastards!'

I had not originally intended a separate chapter on men, but it quickly became clear from the interviews that women had strong views on men, that they had not been able to voice before. When I asked the first woman, by chance, what she thought of men, she snorted, before composing herself for a long tirade against the gender. And she had described herself as happily married!

I ended up with many questions for this chapter. As older women married for life, what if they chose badly, or the man turned out to be unsuitable? What happened if they were not sexually compatible? How did they perceive men, did they like them, socialise with them as friends? What happened at divorce or widowhood, did they seek new partners? How did they feel about men as opposed to women, did they have them as friends? Did women always have relationships with men of their own age, or did they prefer older or younger men? How did men treat them as older women, did they still come on to them?

There was a deep, untapped well of resentment in older women that their lives had been taken so much for granted by men. This stretched from fathers, to brothers, to husbands. Now widowed, it was looking back on lives devoted to the service of men that made them angry. Looking at their children and grandchildren's lives made them realise what might have been, that they could have lived happier lives. I was not expecting this wave of anger from a generation that has largely come to terms with themselves as women – but it was a common streak running through many conversations. One woman, still married to a man who has led her a miserable dance for all her married life has only just begun, at seventy-seven, to listen to the records that she likes, rather than always submitting to her husband's tastes.

Over and over again, women felt that men of the older generation were only looking for a housekeeper and regular sex. They felt foolish at having put up with such bad treatment for so long. Many referred to their mothers and grandmothers and the terrible things they had had to suffer.

There is always plenty of comment from younger women in the media complaining about men and relationships, but these older women astonished me with their clear analysis of the failings of men. They felt they were the last generation to have to put up with such callous indifference from men, and it seemed that they wanted to bear witness to what had happened, not just for themselves, but for all the generations of women that had gone before. One woman mentioned that she saw herself as the last in a long line of skivvies, a vanishing breed of slaves. They looked back at history with shame and anger. But they also looked forward, to the rising generations who were not living the same lives. They were immensely proud of their daughters and granddaughters who were unwilling to put up with the same treatment and who made demands on their husbands. Several women mentioned that they were delighted to have lived long enough to see a world for women that their mothers could not even have imagined.

Women in their fifties thought men played games. They still categorised women (e.g. fluffy blonde, spinster, hard worker) and were confused when women moved categories. Some women played on the dizzy blonde image to get what they wanted from men socially or at work.

While they felt enormous resentment towards men generally, many of the older generation got on well with men as individuals, often preferring their company to the company of women. But some women saw men as a strange, alien breed; they preferred to stay in the feminine world and didn't have men as friends.

Listening to older women, I wondered where the blame lay. If men were inconsiderate and brutal, why and how had they changed in so short a time? Did part of the fault lie with women themselves, who raised generation after generation of men with the same attitudes?

In less than thirty years, the climate between the sexes has changed completely, and while there may still be room for negotiation in the frostier areas, the fact that the sexes can hold a dialogue at all shows just how radical the changes have been.

The loosening of social bonds has made us more individual. We no longer do as we are told by the establishment, church or neighbours. Indeed the establishment itself is crumbling, with Royal separations, members of the government caught with their trousers down and churchmen questioning the articles of faith. While it's certainly true that politicians have always had affairs, the difference now is that we know about it, and they can no longer feed us the same moral guff without appearing hypocritical. Ministers behaving badly underlines their normality, the Them and Us society; where they told us what to do and we followed obediently, disappears. Of course this also has problematic repercussions – where does the moral lead come from in society? And how can a society of individuals work?

But for women, the resulting importance given to individual happiness has meant liberation from the social ties that have bound them for centuries. While that freedom initially made men uncomfortable, because the previous entrenched positions had been lost, their children were raised in a different spirit. This has meant that the generation of men in their twenties and thirties have different expectations of women, which in turn allows women space for their own lives. This new balance is not achieved without pain on both sides; serious readjustments are required that make women as well as men uncomfortable, but when the alternative is the brutal relationships of the past, we surely have no choice.

The women admired their daughters and granddaughters, but they also thought well of younger men. They felt that the rising generation of men could express their feelings, show affection and seemed to behave in a way to their women that older women envied. This led some of the women interviewed to have affairs with younger men, to tap into what might have been. They showed great faith in the future that relations could and were changing between the sexes in a positive way.

Spanning the generations in these interviews made it clear how much women of my generation take for granted. The liberation of women has also allowed men to change. Our grandmothers wouldn't recognise our open, easy friendships with men, and our sexual freedom and financial independence. Even if many of us complain that men are not perfect, that they don't wipe the table down when they do the washing up, listening to the older women in this group, it became clear that their husbands didn't even know where the kitchen was!

Mavis

Seventy-three. She is now widowed but she was happily married and still considers herself very much in the running for other relationships. She had an affair with a forty-four year old recently which she found delightful.

Men? On the whole, most of them are pigs aren't they! To tell you the truth, they're selfish and lazy. I notice good-looking men in the street, I'm still aware of them, the Peter Bowles type – tall, smart men. Men always treat me with respect.

Women today are much more determined about what they want. They're not just prepared to lie on their back and say get on with it, hurry up. Women today want a little bit more. At one time, it was the men that had all the running, if you didn't take your knickers off and go to bed they wouldn't see you any more. Girls don't care about that now. There's plenty of men round the corner.

When you're a widow, some men assume you're available. It's happened to me twice. Once a neighbour that I knew vaguely had done me a good turn, so I invited him in for a drink. We chatted about this and that and then he put his glass down and said would I like to go to bed now! I said, 'No I would not, thank you very much', the cheek!

Then another time, a friend I hadn't seen in years, a doctor, knocked at the door one day. I was naturally pleased to see him and invited him in. We got talking and he said he supposed I was lonely since my husband died and if I was interested he would be willing. I had to laugh at that one, he just came straight out with it!

Mavis is pleased that her daughter's and granddaughter's generation don't have to put up with the sort of treatment she knows many of her peers have over the years. Women used to be dependent on men for several reasons – both financially and if they got pregnant. The pill has changed all that; women have more control over their fertility.

The attitude of some men to widows surprised Mavis; that men should assume she was available and desperate for sex since her husband died. It's significant that it was men of her own generation who assumed this about her; they were still playing by the old rules, believing that women are not free agents, but need to be approached and persuaded into bed. I'm sure both of them got short shrift from Mavis!

Joan

Fifty-two. She is celibate because of her strong religious beliefs. Her job in local government planning brings her into daily professional contact with men at all levels of the social hierarchy.

I feel men don't understand me and my decision to be celibate. I guard myself a lot, perhaps I don't handle things very well. Where I haven't been upfront soon enough, it's been difficult. With Bill – this man I was interested in who was not a Christian – I can't remember how it came up but we were talking about basic values in life and I said it then. He was very surprised and didn't understand. He had some sort of spiritual background himself though. I had made assumptions about what he understood about my position which were wrong – I hadn't been clear enough about what I felt.

I have men friends, but not many, just a few, fewer now than I did. They are different in outlook, in every way really. The men I talk most deeply with now are family members, that reminds me that in reality we are all people and there is a danger in viewing them as too different.

It was a disappointment to my father, who died fifteen years ago now, that I didn't marry. My mother has supported me very much and been very pleased that I'm happy. So it was a simple acceptance on her part, and in fact in latter years she thought that I would be very foolish to give up all I have.

Joan's strong belief in sex only after marriage makes modern relationships tricky. As she said, at what point do you tell a man you're dating that you are not going to bed with him? It also highlights that assumptions about women have changed radically in the last thirty years with the availability of the pill. In the past, women could give the excuse that they didn't want to sleep with a man because they might get pregnant. When that excuse was removed, women saw it initially as a great freedom from worry, but feminists are now beginning to question a freedom that obliges women to be sexually active. Just because they can, does it mean they have to or want to?

Katherine

Fifty-three. She is in a difficult phase of her marriage. Questions in her marriage have been raised by her new responsibilities at work. She is taking a long look at the values she has lived by up to now.

I do like men but I despise them as well! I pride myself on liking women and the company of women and I do, but I do get a buzz out of having men around as well. They're different and there is the frisson of possible attraction and I just find them great fun. But I think of women in a very different way. We share things that men will never know about and we can be much more raunchy than we can be with men. 'New man' just makes me giggle because does he think he's fooling anybody? All he wants is to get the knickers off!

I despise them because of their attitudes to women, their blindness about women and their reluctance to change, and I feel sad for them, too, because they box themselves into such a corner and they can't get out, no matter how hard they try, they're stuck there.

Men are mostly scared stiff of women, which is possibly

why they're so bad about them. Most men still are afraid of the women they were brought up by and it's transferred to the women they associate with later on.

Men generally treat me as a fluffy little blonde, and I have to say I don't try and disabuse them of of this! I can give the impression of being a fluffy blonde very early, it does get one some places, although at the heart of me I think 'You hypocrite, you're not really like that. I'd like to snap his head off as soon as look at him and he's a silly old fart', but you can't.

Older men are very avuncular to me, invariably they're not that much older than me, but they seem to think of themselves as being older and able to give me a pat on the head and what a pretty little thing. I find it very useful, a lot of my job depends on charming people.

Charm, personality, some indefinable spark is what attracts me. If somebody likes you, you automatically start to like them. The person that I'm absolutely mad about, the one I fancy like mad at the moment, is like my husband was ten years ago, which is interesting.

The notion of any man treating this competent manager as a fluffy little blonde is extraordinary. But there is a double bind here; Katherine knows full well she is nothing of the sort and so lures men into a false sense of security into doing what she wants. It's an age-old trick that has been transferred from the home to the work place. But even if it works, shouldn't Katherine be able to compete as herself rather than using the Stone Age School of Charm Rule Book? And how will things change unless women like Katherine metaphorically kick these men in their goolies?

Brenda

Fifty-four. She has a happy marriage with a strong sexual attraction to her husband. She is nervous of appearing boring in her contentment.

Men frustrate me because they don't act like women basically! They don't see something needs to be done – a woman can see it, it's so obvious. They're too interested in their image and their status. I only have men friends that belong to women friends. I seem to extract cuddles from most men, like a boss I used to work with – if he greets me, he'll always give me a cuddle, I quite like that.

I have a problem with the ideal type. We went on a course here and all the people in the group had to say who they fancied. There were eight of us, and they wanted us to say who we liked as a sort of role play exercise to break the ice. I was the oldest and I didn't know what to say. I'd seen someone on the telly I thought looked quite nice, so I thought I'd better say something, so I said him. I even forget his name now and I thought 'Well that will let me off the hook'. I don't fancy anyone else really other than my husband. He's a gentle man and I suppose I can't see that in other people.

Brenda gives off strong signals of being a happily married woman and men can read the 'keep off' sign. They reassure themselves that she is still a woman by responding to her as if she were their mother; they give her a hug. How different to their reaction to Katherine. The signals are so slight we probably don't even know that we're giving them out, but men are receiving them loud and clear. The way Brenda described the role play incident made me giggle; think of a man, any man, and Brenda thinks of her husband (which is great) and then feels a bit of a nerd.

Marjorie

Seventy-six. She is keen to dispel the myth that sex only arrived in Britain in the sixties. She is disappointed in what she sees in the younger generations sexually.

The art of it with men when I was younger was to hint at the possibility, without giving the impression. It's a lovely game, great fun while it lasted. There were plenty of methods. We used condoms, they were the safest, but there were pessaries too, they were very good. When the war came, my whole group of friends were all very alarmed because we said, 'Oh God, now we're going to have to use British products', because all the best products were made in Germany. But they just changed the names and they reappeared in the shops very quickly.

I don't think much of men. I've never felt unequal. Men are stronger, they have different attributes. I don't say that because he's a man, I'm not his equal, I am. They have to accept me as I am in that respect. I get on with men quite well.

I still see men I fancy in the street sometimes, not often because men today don't take care of themselves. They're so casual with everything, they have no finesse, no subtlety. Younger men think they know it all and they don't. If I were much younger I've often thought I could visualise one of them and say 'Come on'. But this generation think let's grab and bump and grind and that's not what it's about. There's a lot of foreplay, and when I say that I don't mean what you probably mean by foreplay. It's a game and you have to play it like a piece of music.

Marjorie feels the ambivalence that many women of her age feel about men. On the one hand, she has always held her own with men and expected to be treated as an equal; on the other hand the younger men she might now be interested in sexually don't come up with the goods, as far as she is concerned. She sees sex as a sophisticated game between two equally capable players and my generation haven't even read the rule book as far as she is concerned.

Elizabeth

Seventy-seven. She has lived with a husband who finds it impossible to show affection and is deeply affected and shocked by his coldness, as much for his sake as for her own.

Men can't express affection. My husband is absolutely horrified that my grandson, aged eighteen, still wants to kiss him goodbye – I mean a peck on the cheek. James was quite convinced that he was homosexual. He was warm and loving and expressing it in that way, but James couldn't accept that – it's all right when they're tiny but not when they get older. I think it's terribly sad, he doesn't have a loving relationship with anybody or anything. It is incredibly Victorian.

I don't think much of men, they're very selfish, very narrow about a lot of things. A lot of them, not all of them and particularly not the younger ones, but a lot of them have got the attitude that the woman is inferior. There's very few of them that would sacrifice themselves for the sake of anybody else. On the whole they're more interested in feathering their own nest than helping anyone else. Some women may feel differently, I would imagine it depends how they have been treated. If they have had a husband who has looked after them and cosseted them a bit, then I expect they think men are wonderful.

Elizabeth has lived with a man for more than forty years who belongs to another century. He's a dinosaur figure, cold and selfish. Elizabeth has come to terms with life through the love and affection she gets from her children and grandchildren. She is positive about younger men and the affection that they can show. This is due in large part to mothers like herself, who taught the next generation of men to show their feelings. I think of Elizabeth every time someone mentions the good old days and think how grateful we should be that his species is becoming extinct.

Judith

Sixty-two. Widowed, she had a happy marriage that she still misses. She is taken aback by the reaction of the different men in her circle to her widowhood.

I honestly don't know why men assume that I'm available, maybe as they see it, I'm the nearest available person. I thought it was rather shocking [*a man's attentions a week after his wife had died*] because he appeared to be so very fond of his wife. I and another colleague were supporting him through his wife's illness, the other colleague more so than me. She also was more available than me in that she hadn't a relationship of any sort at the time so why did he come to me? I was quite happy to support him and be a friend to him, but I couldn't be after that.

At first he didn't believe me, kept persisting and calling around and I really had to be very, very unkind, very brutal in the end, before he got the message and then he seemed to start mourning after that, oddly enough.

I like men, I do, not men *per se*, but I think there are lots of men I admire just as there are lots of women I like. Men treat me well. I can imagine having a relationship with a younger man, probably more so than with an older man. I've tended to fall for younger men in the past, and I've always tended to appear younger than I am, emotionally I never seemed to be my age. Perhaps I am now, but I didn't seem to be in the past and I just seemed attracted to younger men.

I can imagine getting involved with a man in his forties but I can't imagine getting involved with a much older man. It's partly sexual, definitely, I suppose there again body image is important to me and I can't imagine falling for an older man's body. My partner would have been seventy this year, which seems incredible. He was eight years older than me but he had the body of a much younger man.

When Judith says that she doesn't like men per se, but likes them as individuals, she is echoing many women of her generation who have got into difficulties with men, both at work and socially. The man who pestered her, even though she was in a relationship, seemed to see her as an easy target because of her quiet exterior. He also confused her role as friend and comforter with the idea of sexual comfort, which has made Judith reluctant to engage in that role again with other men. It's as though we need a list of terms of engagement when having any friendships with some men, they don't only mistake our signals, they speak a code from a different planet.

Evelyn

Fifty-six. She has had a non-live-in relationship with the same man for twenty years. They meet on Saturdays and garden, eat, watch telly and sleep together and then he goes home to his mother during the week. She likes the mix of companionship and independence.

Some men treat me like an aunt, some of them treat me like a sister, some of them treat me like a mother, some of them treat me like a child, depending on the age group that I'm mixing with. In the same way as your girlfriends are a part of a pattern in your life, so your men friends are and that, I might add, is one of the nicer things about getting old. You can have 'men friends' and you can count the husbands or companions of your girlfriends as men friends as well.

You don't have that separation of the sexes as you get older, probably because the girlfriends, like myself I suppose, having got a partner, haven't the same fear that they might be attracted to someone different. The competition between the sexes disappears as you get older, in theory, it probably doesn't in practice, but to my observation it appears to be much more relaxed.

When men flirt with me, I laugh at them really, enjoy the joke. I can't say I've had that many propositions really [*she laughs*], not recently. Some men do it because it's second nature to them, in the same way as some women cannot walk into a room where there's several people without drawing attention to themselves. Some men flirt because it's a habit and if you took them up on it, they'd be the most alarmed of the lot you know.

Evelyn shows that women in their fifties have taken choices in types of relationship that were just not open to women a generation before. She has an ongoing relationship with a man, but retains her independence and wants to keep it that way. Evelyn has always felt easy in the company of men, coming from a large family, she was used to the rough and tumble of relationships.

Clare

Fifty-six. Her husband is in bad health and they no longer have a sexual relationship. She is fiercely loyal and supportive of him, but aware of the difficulties of not having a sexual relationship when she still feels a strong sexual identity.

I do like men. I have close men friends. Not having a sexual relationship with my husband hasn't put me off men, not at all! I suppose with men I have more of a casual relaxed relationship. Women are more serious, maybe competition comes into it, backbiting, that sort of thing. Men tend to be friends to both of us, I wouldn't see them on their own. I like younger men, certainly they seem to have different attitudes to relationships and to marriage. I do envy that.

For a younger woman, Clare has old-fashioned views about the relations between the sexes. She sees women as the opposition, as competition. It's the old divide and rule approach, which suits the male world very well. This is reinforced by her view of men as a threat or somehow magical, she wouldn't dream of having men friends on her own as she would see a sexual implication there. The outcome is that women like Clare are caught in a world of isolation – women are potential rivals and not to be trusted and men are only after one thing. The subtext to this world view is that you must cleave to your husband, forsaking all others.

Caroline

Seventy-three. She is a woman's woman, a Woman's Institute woman. She has had complicated marriages, but has now remarried her first husband after a difficult divorce.

On the whole I get on better, more easily with women. I suppose I'm a little bit shy of men really. I've got quite a few men friends who are husbands of my women friends but I haven't struck out and found any particular men myself. I don't particularly feel the need for men. The things that I like doing seem to involve women rather than men. It doesn't bother me that I don't have any particular men friends. I think I find women easier to get on with.

Although nearly twenty years older than Clare, Caroline has interpreted the rules differently. She sees herself operating very much in the feminine world, without seeing men as the enemy or being threatening in any way. This is partly because of the hobbies that interest her, which are largely feminine, but also as a result of her world view – she is self-contained in a way that many men would find daunting. And she is immediately appealing to women, we have lots to chat about straight away, she's one of those people you feel you have known for years.

Alice

Sixty. She has had two marriages with people she describes as wasters. She is now living with her first husband who has saddled her with a pile of debts. She resents not being taken care of by men, though she is boss of her own company. There is the paradox of her being extremely capable and efficient and wanting to be taken care of.

Men are bastards! They're weak, not as strong as women, very much the weaker sex in every single way. Men are frightened of me now because I'm strong. I don't think there is anyone out there for me, in fact I'm positive about that. Men are weak and shits, they really are. Men need strong women, there are no strong men, I swear to you there are no strong men! I don't think there are any reliable men out there! I've never looked for a man, they just appear. I'm surprised at really attractive, younger girls who haven't got a fella, why? It's crazy. Men have always found me, I've never done the chasing.

My first husband, I didn't know him, I knew of him, I knew there was this bloke that all the girls thought was fantastic. He was the greatest catch in the area. Another friend said would I go for a drink in this pub, because this particular bloke would like to meet me – he picked me out. That was very flattering. The second one, I was going on holiday with a girlfriend and I had a passionate romantic interlude with the courier. I was very much over the top really, but they picked me out every time. When I got back, I went to a restaurant club and I was with the girlfriend and I went to play the one-armed bandit and someone said try these for luck. It was a bag of threepenny pieces and that was my second husband.

I love the company of men, I flirt. I prefer the company of men to women. Flirting is about self-esteem, someone is telling you by flirting that you are attractive. I'd never start the flirting in case I got rebuffed. I can flirt over the telephone as well. I don't flirt because I think it's going to lead to anything – if I thought it was, I'd run the other way. They used to call me a prick teaser, that's probably what I am. I've never made a play for a man. It's like the no-hopers are homing in on me!

Alice shows what happens when the signals between the sexes get completely muddled. She loves the company of men but has an uncanny knack of picking out the joker in the pack. I suspect that she doesn't really like men or understand them. She chooses what she refers to as the wasters and no-hopers and then expects them to become responsible and take care of her. She's an old-fashioned girl who plays to men's weaknesses and would love to relinquish her strength and capabilities into the arms of a man with a solid bank balance.

Madeleine

Seventy-three she has a rock-solid, happy marriage. They met and danced together and from the moment they first touched they knew it was right. In separate conversations, both describe feeling the same way still about each other. She found her beauty as a younger woman could be a handicap and has found menopause and getting older a relief in many ways.

I like men, but they're very immature as a group, they don't grow up as women do. There are some very special ones, but in general they just move from mother to wife and clean shirts. They don't take their place in looking after the children. That is what makes a woman mature, the responsiblity of the family.

In a way menopause was a relief because I was very pretty when I was young and I had a lot of attention from men, which wasn't always welcome. Menopause gave that feeling of 'Gosh, I can really relax I'm not going to be desirable anymore!' [*She laughs.*] The skin goes and the sag starts, not that I put on a lot of weight or anything like that, it's just that feeling, 'Ah well, I'm not that young woman anymore'. Of course you don't change from one day to the next and I found that I still seemed to be attractive to people, so it didn't just switch off. It's certainly a relief to think that you might not have that attention. Men that you meet are really just friends, there aren't any sexual overtones which there had been. I always mostly worked with men, for eleven years I worked in industry, and however businesslike it all is, there are just those innuendoes that creep in. But I feel now I can deal with men on an even footing.

Madeleine feels that getting older has given her a welcome mantle of invisibility, she can move among people without being judged purely on appearance.

Jenny

Fifty-four. She has been getting over a divorce and sorting out, through therapy, a relationship with a cruel, undemonstrative mother. She has begun dating again and is bemused by what she has found in her various encounters.

I've mixed with quite a lot of men in their fifties and sixties recently and on the whole they are looking at younger women, it's a boost to their egos. Some are quite surprising; I nearly had the clothes ripped off my back once. He was sixty-five and I hadn't been expecting it at all, no way. I'd already met him several times and I went back to his flat. We'd been out to lunch and he said, 'Right let's go to bed'. I told him I hadn't come there for that and he got very frenzied and angry, so I just thumped him one – not hard, just shoved him and told him he was a dirty old man!

He looked a bit ashamed and I left. It was the last thing I ever expected from him as he was a stalwart of the church. I've had two lunatics. The other one I met from an ad in the paper. I don't go out with them straight away, I do chat to them for a long time on the phone first and meet somewhere very public and just chat and make acquaintance. Anyway, I met this man for the second time and he told me he was about sixty-two. I thought he looked older. This second time, we went for a drink in a pub and he said he had been married during the Second World War. So I did my sums and worked out he must be about seventy-two. And then he said, 'When do you want to go away for a dirty weekend!' I said I didn't, that is not the intention of meeting anyone.

Then I thought I'd had enough, so I said goodbye and went out to my car and he shoved me against a shop doorway. He put his hand straight up my skirt and grabbed hold of me and stuffed his tongue straight down my throat! And he was seventy-two!

I was nearly sick. I kneed at him and got in the car and came home. I laugh now, but it was horrid at the time. But it also shows tremendous disrespect, that this is what women are looking for. We had spent some time together, after all, and I'm obviously not that sort of person. He'd been fine the first time, I'd spent the day on the beach and he had even invited my daughter along – and suddenly to do that.

The most amazing thing was that he still got back in touch with me, phoned me up several times as if he had done nothing wrong! Whether he thought that is what women expected, that's what he had to do, I don't know. A man that old would put me off and the very reason it puts me off is from the sex angle – I'll be honest about it. I suppose I think sex stops at seventy! He probably wouldn't be able to manage it and we wouldn't have a proper satisfactory sexual relationship and I would want that.

Jenny is back on the dating game, but the rules don't seem to be clear. Men of a certain age are confused by signals of friendship or interest into thinking that they must make what they would call 'a pass'. And pass is just what Jenny wants to do with men who lunge.

Sally

Fifty-two. She has rediscovered her sexuality at menopause after years of bringing up children single-handed. She has found younger men attractive and attracted. She has never slept with anyone older than herself and believes that younger men pose no danger of real commitment.

I wish someone would send me a list of men around my age! I don't wish them to be beautiful, but I would like them to have the strength and optimism of the women I know. Part of the rage is that you see men who act out the younger women thing. Older men blatantly being applauded for marrying younger women, running off with au pairs. Whereas, with a few exceptions, the toy boy – which is a horrible term – the taking on of a younger man on a full-time basis doesn't happen a lot to women. My rage is double, I see men with younger women, while I myself, because of respect for younger men, would not do that, although I might go to bed with them. Therefore we have been left high and dry, that is the rage. Older men aren't interested in us, they call us batty, scatty old women and names like that. It's a self-fulfilling prophecy, if you're made to feel like a second-class citizen, you become one.

I had a very bad relationship with my father, so I don't have much respect for men, I feel safer living on my own. I would swap one good man for all the affairs I've had, most of which were inconsequential. In theory, I like the idea of having a man around, I would like that a lot, but I don't seem to be programmed for it.

If you feel uncomfortable and ill at ease with men and have always felt like that, then it makes it difficult. However, younger men seem to be attracted to me at the moment and I can't deny there is something deeply flattering about that. There's a seemingly endless supply of younger men!

Sally is confronting a problem that affects many women of her age, the fact that older men largely seem to be interested in younger women. Menopause has made her feel rage at the situation older women are caught in. Yet, paradoxically, she also finds herself attracted to younger men who are clearly responding to her. She also separates bed from real relationships, a divide that strikes me as rather too surgical. She veers from respect for younger men to a more predatory attitude, highlighting her own uncertainty about relationships.

Maud

Seventy-eight. She is widowed after a happy marriage. She is a strong woman who would like a dinner companion or someone to go on holiday with but definitely not a live-in man.

I like a certain kind of man – intellectual. I don't like the crowd that get together at the pub, talking football and women, I can't stand that lot. But I like serious intellectual men, who give me the respect of wanting to know what I really think. But there's absolutely no sexual attraction anywhere. I haven't got a lot of female friends, although I have a lot of acquaintances. I've never found many women that I've got this intellectual thing with, not many of them want to talk in depth about anything very much. In fact, I feel I put a lot of people off by suddenly launching into a subject and they brush it aside and they don't want to know about it.

Maud has always been attracted by intellectuals, but has also been plagued by women believing she is trying to get off with their partners. If a woman takes on the male (so called intellectual) agenda, particularly in a social situation, then she takes on male attributes (forceful, with opinions) and yet is accused of trying to seduce those men. I can imagine a woman like Clare being terrified of Maud speaking to her husband at a party. In her world view, women are supposed to be receptors, to reflect and applaud the male agenda. And they are then selected by the men for their femininity, their passive docility.

Dot

Seventy. She had a disastrous first marriage with a man she describes as a psychopath, followed by many affairs and then a happy, stable marriage for twenty-five years. Crisis at menopause prompted deep questioning and therapy. She is now a counsellor herself and optimistic about life for the first time.

I do like men, very much indeed. But I like women better! I do not trust men still and I certainly love women, there is a bond and a friendship between women which supersedes any thing with men. Once you realise men are from a different planet and respect them for that, everything becomes clear. They do not speak our language. But I do like men and get on with them well.

After many years of chasing the wrong men, Dot has come to terms with them. She has realised that she doesn't need to sleep with them to get affection, and that the fact that they march to a different drummer doesn't mean she can't play in the same band.

Chapter Five

Celibacy

Most of us will be celibate at some time in our lives, from choice or obligation, whether in relationships or not. Most relationships go through celibate patches; in the normal rhythm of a long-term commitment, it would be surprising if they did not. The stresses of modern life, illness, long hours of work, or simply not fancying the partner for a while mean that many couples go for weeks or months without having sex. Those not in relationships may feel they have no choice but to be celibate and may be concerned that the breather between relationships may go on longer and longer. But many people choose to be celibate. The religious life often calls people to celibacy or is seen in some religions as an ideal to which they should aspire.

So why, if so many of us are celibate at one time or another in our lives, is it not more openly discussed, rather than being treated like an infectious disease? And if that seems a bit strong, when was the last time someone told you they were celibate?

Sex permeates our lives; from ice cream advertisements to prostitute cards in telephone booths, from tabloid shockers to double entendres at work. So what are we getting so worked up about? Commercially sex sells. The pillar of society caught with his trousers down appeals to the prurient in us all, the religious freak who kidnaps the object of her passion and chains him to her bed has us all roaring with laughter. Advertising uses sex, more or less subtley, to tempt us; buy this ice-cream, car, new gadget and the opposite sex will run up to you with a bunch of flowers, fall headlong at your feet, find you irresistible.

It all boils down to fear – the fear is of being alone, being unwanted, being celibate. In France, it's not so long since spinsters were singled out by being addressed as 'Mademoiselle' even in their seventies. The implication was that they had failed in finding a mate and were therefore not to be graced with the more respectful 'Madame'. One woman I know in France turned this to good effect; having been left at the altar by her prospective husband, she never married and insisted on being called Mademoiselle by all and sundry to emphasise the wrong done to her.

In this chapter, I wanted to look at how older women felt about celibacy. We tend to assume that the older women get, the more likely they are to be celibate. The younger you are, the younger you place the cut-off point (remember how in your twenties you couldn't imagine people in their forties having sex!), and as you approach middle age it tends to be about fifteen years older than your own age. Of course, each time you approach that notional barrier, you may find you want to push it on another fifteen years!

I wanted to find out from older women if they were celibate whether or not they were in relationships. How did they cope with being left or losing their partners? What of women who were celibate through choice, for religious or other reasons? How did women cope with celibacy, did they masturbate or fantasise or find other outlets? How did they set about finding partners if they felt they wanted sex? Did they feel that they had been more celibate round menopause, or was it a time of enhanced sexuality with all those hormones whizzing round?

Some women in their seventies and eighties, who had never had good sexual relationships, were glad to have an excuse to finish with 'all that business'. If they were married to older men, their husbands often had health problems which made sex difficult, if not impossible. Many of them reported feeling additional closeness if sex was no longer possible. It seemed to allow space and time for cuddles and affection. Many women at menopause had problems with dry vaginas, and for some sex became too painful.

Younger women in their fifties and sixties often mentioned being bored with their partners if they were married. They fantasised about other men, but were often reluctant to put thought into action for fear of disrupting the status quo. Others used periods of celibacy to stimulate desire, a couple of weeks with no sex and both husband and wife were enthusiastic again. Others again used periods of enforced celibacy, brought on by death or divorce, to reconsider their lives before jumping back into sexual relationships.

Our society has an Ark mentality – if we're not two-by-two we're afraid that we might not be admitted. The reinforcement from our family and peer group is astonishingly strong; women reported people trying to match-make them with completely unsuitable men. It seemed any man would be better than no man at all – complete no-hopers were pulled out of the cupboard, dusted down and given another airing at excruciating dinner parties.

The rise of the dating agency, with the enticing couples smiling coyly from newspaper ads, reinforces the message that if you are on your own, there must be something wrong with you, somehow it is your own fault. Women who tried them reported varying success, with the men you wouldn't touch with a barge pole outweighing the possibles by a huge factor.

It's time to challenge the stereotype of the sad old maid, and regard celibacy as a sabbatical from the humdrum of sexual relations. Women particularly need time for themselves, for their own needs, which can easily become obscured by the demands of the myth of the modern Superwoman who works, looks after her family, cooks cordon bleu meals and is a wow in bed. No wonder she looks a bit frayed round the edges. For women on their own, it's difficult to resist the pull of couple power, it's so much easier to slide back into the norm. But relationships are not card tricks; pick a man, any man, and you're likely to end up with a disaster. Being alone gives time for reflection, time to spend on yourself at last.

It's a useful exercise to look around the people you know and try and guess how many of them are going through a celibate patch. It's a fair bet that a high percentage of people, in or out of relationships are celibate. And if you don't believe that coming out as a celibate is like admitting to a bad case of leprosy, try asking them.

Katherine

Fifty-three. She has been married for many years, without a very satisfactory sex life. While talking about celibacy in her marriage, she comes to some startling conclusions. We spend some time later discussing the consequences.

Most of the time, I have been disappointed with sex in our marriage. At the moment we're trying a bit of celibacy. It might be that we're not sexually compatible, or maybe it's because we set up the wrong rules at the beginning. We were so inexperienced, in those days one was. But there's a great deal of love there, so that surely should take you through.

I'm very, very busy, working hard all day and then travelling home. I just can't be bothered to make an effort really. It's just developed in the last few months, whether it will go on or not, I don't know. Working has liberated me sexually, too, but not in order to go and have affairs. Having this period of celibacy is my way of coping with the changes that have to be made. Thinking about it and talking about it like this makes me realise it's like stop, take a deep breath and look at what's happening, without the old habits. Maybe that is the way to do it.

Sexual compatibility can be worked on, but whether it's too late for us now, I don't know. I've thought about going to 'masterclasses', it sounded rather funny, when you hear people relating their experiences. By and large, we come from a generation that doesn't believe in that kind of thing. It's self-indulgence and we think you must sort it out for yourself, but if it goes on too long I suppose that would be the only way to bring it back.

It'll need me to sit down and face it. I'm going to have to initiate a discussion of some kind and I'm avoiding that, it's very hard, especially when you're an avoider like I am. I'm an 'I'll talk about it later' sort of person, but I'll have to do it. It has to be me, because I probably wouldn't listen to him, he wouldn't be able to pin me down well enough now. There's never a good moment, I've come up to appropriate moments a couple of times and not taken the step, so I'm going to have to decide. Some of my colleagues are so bloody organised, they plan their lives to the day and say, 'Next week, I'm going to do so and so'. That's what I'm going to have to do.

Also, it's almost embarrassing to think of something sexually different. If you're ever watching a soap opera and two of the characters kiss, it's sort of ooh, embarrassing. That's the feeling I would get, I'd have to be really pissed to do something radical. We've never talked about it, that's another thing, communicating about this is very difficult, the embarrassment factor sets in.

I shall have to see, after this period of celibacy, if it's something that's very serious in our relationship or whether we can just weather it. In a marriage as long as mine, there are bound to be times when one person is not in tune with the other. In the past, there have been times when it's been almost mutual, because we just simply haven't liked each other very much. I can't recall for the life of me what brought it back again. It's happened a couple of times.

When Katherine talks about her husband, to whom she has been married for so long, in some ways she is talking about a stranger. Their lack of communication in sexual matters is now so well established that it seems an impossible pattern of silence to break. But he also seems unable to communicate his vulnerability at having lost regular work, so their sexual difficulties have become a wrestling point between them. Katherine sees celibacy as a breather, a chance to take stock and move on to a more positive scenario, the danger being that celibacy will become a negative habit that will be even more difficult to talk about or emerge from. She sees it very much as her role to try and break them out of this impasse, perhaps if she could give him some of the responsibility for communication, things might change. Katherine prefers to avoid the subject, in the hope that it will go away or be forgotten about, but what they really need is to start talking, even if it is just about the characters kissing in Coronation Street.

Joan

Fifty-two. She has thought deeply about the issues surrounding celibacy and their implications for her life. She is the least likely person you'd pick out in the crowd as being celibate.

I do believe, without being fatalistic, that God does have some plan for our lives. I long ago said, 'Lord if you want me to be married, that would be just great with me, but if you don't, then that's fine too'. I'm not sure whether I expected Him to take me up on it, but looking back I think He has. It's something I have to trust Him with. Also I don't think it's the be all and end all of life.

Pressure from all around could lead one to question one's identity without *it*, because *it* assumes such large proportions. I'm not saying that it's always been easy, but I do think every role or every path in life has opportunities and constraints. Our natural tendency is to want to experience everything, certainly where sex is concerned as there's such a mystique surrounding it, and one wouldn't be human if one didn't have curiosity or desire to experience.

Being celibate has been a choice, basically because of my spiritual convictions. I became a Christian when I was eighteen, and certainly I had quite strong convictions about God's purpose for us in the context of marriage and His view of our bodies.

I am firmly of the opinion that sex is intended for marriage, and is entirely good and healthy and everything else, but that it is intended for a one man, one woman relationship. The body, in Biblical terms, is intended to be the temple of the Holy Spirit, which is terribly technical talk, but that is how it is described. I believe that God has rules for us, which I can understand some people might see as inhibiting, but I can only say that personally I have sought to abide by what I saw as God's good plan. That's why I have not had sex, because I've not been married.

I don't think I had that much understanding of the situation when I became a Christian when I was eighteen. I joined a Bible study group and I very soon began to realise that this was God's pattern and I assented to it. At the time I was involved in quite a conservative group, which I must say was a strong influencing factor on me. So the very group membership applied a certain constraint on me. Of course, later I moved away from that, although I still continue to be involved in a church and with the same people. But the sort of constraint one experiences at the age of eighteen, through a peer group, falls away and one has testing times.

It has been difficult at times, but I don't think it's so much being unsure of my decision, it's been a failure to communicate well enough in the relationship which has been very complicated. I'm conscious that because it's not the norm, that if one is to have an honest relationship, one has to be very honest about this.

There's been a fear on my part that if a man knew I wasn't going to go to bed with him, that that would be it. Of course that's a risk that one would have to run, but it's a difficult one, because it's hard to know when to make this statement.

I wouldn't say I'm not affected by celibacy, I wouldn't say that. There have been times when I've struggled with it, because we do have physical drives within us, particularly if we are fond of people and in a relationship. There's a natural desire to express oneself physically, to communicate physically and I have found that to be quite a battle at times. It's a battle that's come and gone. I don't mean by that that it's over, it's cyclical.

But then again, if I go back to my spiritual foundations, I find that there is truth in the fact that whatever we feed, grows. If I allow myself to be preoccupied with watching and thinking and reading forever about things to do with sex, then it affects me, and makes life more of a struggle. Without being escapist, I have determined in my life that I want to give my energies to positive things. One of the decisions I made long ago was how I wanted to relate to people. I really wanted, and still want, to be the sort of person who gives to other people. By doing that, it takes the focus off one's own needs. Of course, it doesn't just apply in this area of life, it applies in all kinds of realms.

I did fall in love with someone who wasn't a Christian . . . I haven't had lots and lots of relationships. I've had friendships with a few men, and there was one particular relationship where it was the biggest struggle of all. That was when things might have . . . if I was ever going to give in to it, it would have been then (when I was forty-five), rather late in life.

I could see that my beliefs did make a difference in the way we made decisions. It made a difference in all kinds of ways. The way we viewed our priorities, the way we spent our time, used our money. It would have made a difference how we viewed and treated people in our home together.

I don't think that could have been resolved because it seemed so fundamental. That all sounds on the negative side. But the other thing is in my relationship with God, it's very important to me, in fact it's at the core of who I am, so if I couldn't really show that with the other person, that would be a great limitation on the relationship.

I would only want to marry a Christian, that's at the heart of it really. I feel that Christian thinking colours my attitudes and my value systems, and that it would be the only foundation on which I would contemplate marrying somebody. Now, of course, there are lots of Christian men around, but I haven't married one of those because the ones I wanted haven't wanted me!

Being celibate gives me a freedom with people that I think I wouldn't otherwise have. It enables me to work with men, with colleagues, it gives me freedom in those terms because it avoids complications, put it that way. It's enabled me to put a lot of energy into my friendships and my work.

I must come over as fairly cool because I'm probably guarding myself. In fact I know I am, and unless men really want to get to know me, they tend to think that I'm a bit distant, so they don't make advances.

Friends used to try and invite me to things and pair me off – I'd meet their brother, or their father, or their son. I always felt very angry with that and wouldn't comply, so that soon stopped. But no, I don't wear a lapel button to say all this and I don't really know whether it comes over to people.

I'm not sure that I would separate sexuality from gender. I'm very interested in womanly things, if I can stereotype a little bit. I enjoy my home enormously – needlework, entertaining, doing things around the place. In my job, I'm head of department and the way I operate is female, and by that I mean I am concerned for people and I am not prepared to be ruthless in some ways that might be expected of me if I don't think that is the appropriate thing to do. Those are my strengths at work, my weaknesses in fact are being aggressive and pushing forward.

I enjoy work, partly because it reinforces who I am, but also because I do enjoy talking to men and hearing their perspectives and having comradeship with them. I try not to flirt with them, I've trained myself to try and think of men as people, as opposed to men! If I'm being honest, I play down that side of things. It's protection of me, I suppose. I find certain men attractive, very, I could tell you from this weekend conference who I think are the really dishy ones.

Joan's decision to be celibate challenges the view that anyone who could have sex would choose to do so. She's an attractive woman who has made celibacy a positive and difficult choice in an age where to be is to be available. If you remove sex from the equation of close relationships with men, Joan has concluded that relationships become impossible. The struggle she had with the one man she grew close to shows that this is not a decision that she had made

*lightly, that it sabotaged a relationship that might well have
worked. When I ask her why she doesn't date Christian men,
with the same views as herself (there are even evangelical dating
agencies) she grimaces and gives the old excuse that she has never
liked the ones that like her. What, no Christian man in Britain
would suit her?*

*While celibacy before marriage is an honourable and difficult
moral choice, in a society that screams sex from every advert, plenty
of people hold her views and still find partners and get married. I
realised during the course of the interview that I have been so
intrigued with the idea of an attractive woman choosing not to have
sex that I have ignored the implications of what she is saying. She
chooses to live alone because she doesn't want relationships with
men, despite her high principles – the issue of sex before marriage is
a convenient red herring.*

Marjorie

*Seventy-six. She confounds the stereotype of the older woman. She
feels she has had at least as much sexual freedom throughout her life
as this present generation. She has strong principles but not of a
straightforward kind.*

I'm celibate now, but it hasn't been difficult. I've got lots
of memories, and if an old friend should come to see me
and say, 'How about it?' well that would be fine, I'm not
worried either way, but old habits die hard. People think
celibacy is dreadful, but that's because they've been
reading the wrong books. They've got the wrong expectations because they've been told the wrong things. I
suspect that the old wives are as alive and kicking as
they ever were. They should have been drowned at birth.
I don't know what the hell you're going to make of all this!

*Marjorie's open marriage means she has had more sexual experience
than many women of her generation. She seems to have slipped*

through the moralistic net and found her own path in life. She has battled against sexual ignorance all her life and when we talk about the subject, she is the only woman in the whole group to engage me in discussion. This is a woman who has lived liberation all through her life and finds it perfectly natural to have done so. She holds the old wives' tales responsible for a lot of the ignorance about sex she has found among younger people.

Annie

Fifty-six. Being gay adds an extra dimension to the celibacy that she has found difficult. The gap between generations of women is underlined more strongly in lesbian sexual politics.

I've been celibate for many years now – about nine years – awful thing to have to admit. My sexual drive has never been very strong, ever, but certainly I feel now as if I have totally lost it. I can't remember what it felt like. I remember sex, I remember feeling sexual, so it happened, but it's like trying to remember pain.

I am sad about that. I was talking to a friend the other day, a little bit younger than me. She said to me, if you'll pardon the language, 'Annie, I've got to a point where I feel as if I just want to fuck everything'. Then she said to me, 'You don't feel like that do you?' I said, 'No I don't'. She said she wished she didn't either, but I said, 'Would you rather feel like me?' We couldn't make up our minds which was worse, to be menopausal and feeling like I do or feeling highly sexed. She's a lesbian too. She's in the awful position of getting very strong sexual feelings and not being able to do anything about it and I feel as if I really ought to be just out there gardening in button-up shoes.

Maybe it's a passing thing, but if I did meet somebody I would be so frightened I wouldn't do anything about it anyway. I do feel as if I will never be in a sexual relationship again, and it does bother me. I feel and have felt that I am a single person. New widows often say this too. It's not that nobody asks you out, people do ask me to supper, but nearly all of my friends have partners. I'm the odd one out, the one that doesn't.

I would like to have someone around. I would and I wouldn't. I've got used to living on my own. I would never want to live with anyone again. I've got used to doing things my own way, if I want to sit on the floor, or fall asleep in front of the television, or eat at four o'clock in the afternoon I can do so.

I've got quite a lot of friends but I do feel increasingly lonely. I don't like feeling as if I have dried up. It's quite a chunk of your life that goes missing, and from my life it's been missing for quite a long time now.

I'm not the sort of person who approaches someone, and that is another problem. I wait till they approach me – this is true of very many lesbians. Not the younger women. For a start, there's the uncertainty that the other person might not be gay. You can't stand in a bus queue and say, 'Hands up all the lesbians!' So in terms of meeting somebody at the office, or at a mixed party, you don't know who is and who isn't. Quite often you can just look and think 'dyke' but you can't always guess. These days it's a little more difficult because young heterosexual women dress very dykey, have all their hair chopped off and wear DMs – you can be very misled.

I go to lesbian clubs, but they tend to be discos and young women. There is an older lesbian network, but I find it difficult. I find an awful lot of backbiting goes on, there's always someone who ends up in tears. I mentioned this to my therapist and she said people who are oppressed always turn and oppress either another group or one another. There is another group but they tend to be totally apolitical, middle class and fuddyduddy. There doesn't seem to be much in the middle for people like me.

It has a lot to do with self-confidence, but how else do

you find somebody? Is this why I'm sitting here, not in a relationship? It's worse for lesbians than straight women, and it gets more and more complicated and difficult as you get older.

I would be dreadfully frightened if someone else came along. I have had the odd offer but I didn't fancy any of them – was it fear that made me feel that way? I am a disaster sexually; I'm not attracted particularly to lesbians, I'm not attracted to older women. What young heterosexual woman is going to walk into my life and pick me up? It must be something to do with non-availability.

If someone did come along, all sorts of awful things would crop up about body image. If I could be sure that initially it was only bed! In my attempts at being heterosexual, bed and relationships were very much separate, I tend not to separate so much with women.

With men it was absolutely destined not to work because I only had sex with men who weren't going to be upset when I decided to push off, which I did fairly rapidly. So that meant it was someone I was not going to get fond of anyway. One was a guy I worked with, one was a guy I went to evening class with, it's so much easier to make a relationship with a man. The other day I was in a bus queue, this young man approached me, albeit he was foreign and said, 'I go home with you' and I said, 'No you don't'. Now no lesbian is ever going to do that to me!

Annie is setting herself up to fail. She only fancies younger, heterosexual women who are safely out of her reach. Her celibacy has become a habit, like a worn pair of slippers that should have been thrown out years ago, but you don't notice the holes until someone else points them out. Going to lesbian groups doesn't seem to work for her, each one brings up problems that she is not happy with. But maybe groups are not the answer for her now, although they might have been when she was coming to terms with her sexuality. Yet at some level, she hasn't accepted the fact that she is gay, still fancying unavailable women and being quite passive about her own sexual identity, wanting someone else to make the first move. She herself links this to the severe depression from which she has suffered for many years.

Elizabeth

Seventy-seven. She has accepted her husband's complete lack of affection with a quiet strength which shames him and his generation.

It's over twenty years since I had any physical relationship. We've got separate bedrooms now because we both sleep badly. Sometimes when I'm awake at night, I almost long for someone to cuddle me and possibly have sex with me, so my desire hasn't completely gone away.

If someone came along who I was attracted to and could give me a warm relationship . . . I might like to have a cuddle with someone else, whether I would go further I don't know – because of the family, that would always override everything.

I suppose I've coped by being busy with other things. More and more I am sure that if we had had a very good physical relationship, then my husband would have been a much healthier, happier man. The very fact of holding himself in all the time has been bad for him. But you see, I have been able to expend my love on the children. I've always had young babies around, I've got one now that is only three months old, my latest granddaughter, and I can sit and cuddle her. Fortunately I don't need an awful lot of sex, but I do need warmth and kindness.

Although Elizabeth has been married for many years and has had children, she has virtually led the life of a celibate. Sex was for having children, not for any pleasure between the couple. Not having sex, when the man decided that was it, was just something to be accepted with some relief. A modern woman would have looked elsewhere or asked for divorce. She's pleased that her children and grandchildren have different lives.

Clare

Fifty-six. She has a second loving marriage fraught with difficulty, but she still speaks of her husband with great loyalty and affection.

Our physical relationship has always been difficult, then six years ago he had a very serious heart attack and we have had no physical relationship since. He's not well enough and on so much medication that he is impotent. He's sixty-two now.

I don't know how I have dealt with it; it hasn't always been easy. In the last few years, I have longed for a relationship and I have been quite worried that I might meet somebody and I don't want to because of Stephen. When he had the attack, they said that with this heart he won't reach sixty, but he has and he carries on. If I had an affair, if I met someone, just to sort out that side of my life, he would be bound to find out, and I would never hurt him.

People of your generation think that you can't have a life without sex. This has worried me actually, because I read various things that say it's not a proper marriage. I feel it's a different one. It's not black and white. The media gives a false impression that everyone out there is having sex and when you are a certain age you have sex so many times a week.

I thank my lucky stars that I haven't tripped over someone else, it would be very complicated. I do love my husband and I am very grateful for that and the way he feels about the fact that he is impotent and that we don't have a physical relationship. He is full of guilt and feels awful about it so we don't discuss it a lot now, it has been accepted.

HRT has made me feel better and it certainly hasn't squashed any sexual feelings I had. I could be very easily aroused by something I hear or something I read, so although things aren't going well with Stephen and I on that score, basically I think I could have another happy relationship.

I've channelled that energy into my children and grandchildren and into work. In a way, I feel inadequate sometimes that maybe I'm different. I think of other women, people in marriages with good sexual relationships, still with their husbands in their fifties, sixties, seventies. Have I missed out all these years?

I don't talk about it with friends, but I've talked about it with my elder daughter and she said, 'I thought that's how it was Mum'. It's not something that has worried me so much that I've felt I needed to talk about it, maybe it would have been good to have had some counselling, I don't know. It helped to talk to my daughter about it.

I do wish things had been different, but I stuck with him. I love him and basically he needs me. If I've noticed men who were attracted to me, I've enjoyed perhaps an evening of chatting to somebody, if we were both attracted to each other. But I'm scared, I don't want to upset the apple cart at the moment, I really don't.

Clare measures her celibacy against the norms she reads about in women's magazines and is worried that her marriage is not a 'proper' one because they can no longer have sex. But the idea of a 'normal' sexual pattern is ridiculous, fed to us by magazines who know good copy when they see it; the 'must have sex twice a week syndrome', because that is the national average, is nonsense. What is important is only what makes both partners happy. Celibacy is perhaps unusual in someone Clare's age, but many women stop having sex when their partners develop health problems. She has recently been thinking ahead to the time when her husband may not be around, putting her sexual life on hold for the moment.

Rose

Eighty-four. She had a long and happy marriage with a husband who had bad health. Life has always been a struggle but there are no complaints. Sex during marriage was more of a chore than anything else, a view held by many of her generation who knew very little about sex before their marriage.

People say to me, 'Why didn't you remarry?' But I'm very independent, I try and do things for myself. If the right man had come along, I believe I would have got married again. I met different people at luncheon clubs, used to dance with them, but it never got any farther than that. There was one man who came and talked to me, he seemed very lonely and he was very shy, but he talked to me and I was only too glad to talk back.

I think you get more sense out of men! We went out once or twice, but it didn't go any farther. I didn't do anything, it's just that terrible shyness from when you are very young, you just can't shake it off, it stays with you. It has to come from the man. I never gave the impression that I felt all that much for this man, he was a friend that was all.

Rose is a product of a different age; when women did not approach men, or let them know they were interested. But she is also very independent and has had to manage a household single-handed, bringing up children and caring for an invalid husband. Rose was brought up to believe that men are the active agents in society and women are passive. Yet she has been active personally and in politics all her life. But though she can happily go on a march for rights for the elderly, she could no more let a man know she was interested than she could fly.

Caroline

Seventy-three. She divorced her first husband and remarried, but she is now married to her first husband again.

My present husband has got a neurological problem that he has had for fifteen years and sex isn't a possibility, but it hasn't worried us. It doesn't worry me in the least now. I haven't had any sex since 1975. I don't miss it at all, although I did a bit to start with.

Caroline has had several periods of celibacy in her life, between marriages, and now a longer spell since her husband's illness. But she has also had good sex with both her husbands, so she knows what she might be missing. The idea that someone might just give up sex may shock a younger generation who often measure their happiness by their sex lives. But as she explained, life has different phases of activity, and what is appropriate to one doesn't hold in the next. She has used celibacy in the past to get on with her career, now it means she has more time and energy for her own needs.

Mavis

Seventy-three. She is attractive and very aware of her sexuality. She has recently finished a delightful affair with a forty-four year old man, but she has by no means discounted the idea of other relationships should they come along.

When my husband died, everything died with him – it was such a shock, he died very suddenly. Sexually I didn't want sex, I didn't even think about it and it didn't worry me. It's a mystery to me, just one of those things. I didn't have a relationship for ten years.

About four years ago I met a young man of forty-four. I had been working and this man said, 'Let's go for lunch'. We went and I can see him now sitting opposite me saying, 'How would you like to have a relationship?'

So I thought, 'Hmm, I want to think about it, am I going to be embarrassed or anything like that?' but I wasn't. I hadn't been with anyone for about ten years. I thought 'Can I still? Will it be all right?' When it was going to happen, I was terrified, what was I going to feel like? I thought I was going to feel terribly awkward. Once it happened, it was fine, absolutely wonderful. In fact it was great, neither of us worried about it, so there were no inhibitions whatsoever. He was married and I started having a sexual relationship and of course people used to say, 'You've got a toy boy!' It lasted about a year, and it was very good, I thoroughly enjoyed it, I would recommend it!

I knew it couldn't last, but it was good for me, very good for me, and I'm sure it was good for him. I don't think my sexual appetite ever depreciated, it was always very good. We always said, you don't fall in love, you get on well.

Age didn't come into it, we'd go out when we were together, it didn't seem to make any difference at all. In fact I think he rather liked it. My daughter thought it was wonderful, she would like me to have another affair! I'm very content the way I am, but if I were to meet someone, it would be fine. I wouldn't put myself out at all to meet someone though.

Mavis surprised me when she told me she'd had an affair with a married man – it wasn't the age gap so much as the fact that I'd expected an older person to be more conservative and play by the rules. When I asked what happened in the end, she told me he did what all married men do; he went back to his wife. Her acknowledgement that the affair was not going anywhere, that they didn't imagine they were falling in love, indicates that Mavis was able to give herself wholly to the immediate moment. I think that's what surprised me too, that she should act 'irresponsibly', again confounding all my prejudices about older women.

Jenny

Fifty-four and divorced. She has had long periods on her own, punctuated by dating different men. She has a teenage daughter still at home, who herself is just beginning to date.

It's a myth that older women are more celibate, definitely, it's one of our closely guarded secrets! I think, 'Ha, ha, they think we're just knitting and have gone past it, and it's not nice in women over fifty'. It's a myth for young people, they think they're the only ones who do it. In the media, older men are sexually active, but not women in their fifties and sixties.

I have had patches of loneliness. Not having anyone around, one thing that has really got to me, made me really low, is the fact that I haven't had any family support, I've had to get on with it on my own. I haven't got a family really; my sister lives on the other side of the world and my two sons are quite slow and backward, so I can't expect support from them, not that you would from sons anyway. Neither of my sons will ever marry and I support them a lot, so I have felt very much alone. My daughter needed me. That's the one thing that has got to me and made me feel very lonely. If I had just a sister in this country that I could have picked up the phone and gone to see, it would have helped.

I've been celibate through circumstance mainly. I've been anxious that this may be it, will I never have sex again, will anybody fancy me? You do think that. I would have been disappointed if that had been it. I don't see celibacy as positive at all, it's not just the sex, it's the closeness and communication, everything that goes with it, just someone to put their arm round you.

If I didn't feel I needed a man, I probably would get on and do things, get a lot more done, but if you still feel you need some sort of sexual fulfilment, life is more complicated. Sexuality is about companionship too. Why do we think of older women as not having sex? Because their bodies change and they get all wrinkled and saggy and look old. You think they wouldn't appeal to anyone, unless it was someone of their own age, or that they wouldn't be at all interested in sex.

I can't imagine that I'll still be having sex in my eighties, though I don't know where the cut-off point is! It's just how you're conditioned – that older women don't, older men do. But life is more than about having a man around. I used my celibacy as a period of healing in a way, making lots of new friends and going on holiday with them. I had to find myself and know what I wanted and know where I was going. I tried to use that time as positively as I could.

I never got used to being celibate. When another man came along I wasn't surprised, I thought 'Things are looking up again!' On to the next patch, I'm better now, because I wasn't really very good company for a long time after the break up of my marriage.

Jenny is in the strange position of starting dating again, at the same time as her fourteen-year-old daughter is beginning to take her first steps in the dating dance. Although she has been married and has grown-up children, Jenny displays many of the worries of the first timer. Will I find anyone? Does he really like me? When should we kiss? Who should make the first move? When her daughter comes home from school, she's worried about a disco that evening. Jenny calms her down and she goes off to do her homework. Jenny says she understands her daughter completely because she feels just the same!

Florrie

Eighty-four. After two happy marriages, though the first was not a sexual success, she now has a live-in boyfriend in his sixties.

I'm not sure it was worth waiting to have sex, not for the man I married. Perhaps if it had been someone worth waiting for, then yes! I wouldn't have married him if I had known that it didn't work, sexually I mean, between us. I definitely think that. I agree with knowing before you get married, finding out what you are letting yourself in for!

The first one, he just wasn't any good at it, he didn't really know what he was doing! This one doesn't either, the man who is living in my house at the moment. The few times we've tried he'd not the slightest idea! I don't mind anymore. I wouldn't bother to teach him better, there's no point, you wait until you get older, you'll see what I mean! A good night's sleep is better than that.

People should sleep together before marriage, it's such a big thing, so important to a relationship, such a big part of marriage. You hear stories that some men are so horrible. Most are hopeless, they just flop like fishes, flounders! There's enough stuff around nowadays, they ought to be able to get some information from books.

Florrie looks back on her first marriage with sadness, but it is only because she had a good sexual experience with her second husband that she then knew that she had missed out. But what of the countless numbers of women who were never lucky enough to have a second chance at sexual happiness? She's someone who has never been on her own for long and clearly inspires devotion in her current live-in boyfriend.

Sally

Fifty-two. She has had many celibate years off and on since the break-up of her marriage twenty years ago. Left with two young children, her sexuality went on hold until menopause.

I've been principally celibate for twenty years and still am. Rationally, what happened completely took me by surprise, which was that I was so terrified of this thing called fifty, I completely forgot about forty-nine. I've been mainly celibate since 1979, with a few one-night stands and a couple of very short, but most unimportant relationships, then I had a relationship with a much younger man which was like a thunderbolt. I was shocked by my physical feelings. The affair wasn't very long and it felt strange. It could have either been the fright of forty-nine or the hormonal change. Things that had been submerged came to the surface. One side of me thought I had always been like that, but my mothering had stopped me letting it out, had squashed my sexual feelings. I had very, very strong sexual feelings, not just the romantic passionate side of it, but a real need for sex.

But I also chose someone who was entirely unsuitable, so therefore it wouldn't proceed. It wasn't a relationship, I've never put all my eggs in one basket, because that would be a real fright, that you would lose yourself.

There was almost a kind of mystical thing about forty-nine. That's the other side, the feeling and intuition that I'd always been like that, a very sexual person, but it hadn't come out.

In a sense, the menopause was releasing something and the hormones do go haywire. So it could be that at certain points you get the rushes of hormones that provoke this feeling of sexuality. Mind you it was provoked though, I didn't go out looking for some young man, the young man approached me. It could have been coincidental. He was twenty-six. Having affairs with young men is safe, whereas a man of my own age would be more dangerous, it scares me because there is more likelihood that something might come of it.

I don't anticipate not wanting to go to bed with people. I once put an ad in the paper, but I got pathetic answers, even though my ad was tremendous. I gave up on that idea. I would like to continue to have sex but I don't know how I'm going to do it. I don't want to have a 'live–in' as I work from home. I find most of the men I meet to be very disappointing on most levels and sex doesn't come through the letter box! Celibacy can be positive for women at some stages. I never said I was going to be celibate. A friend of mine said she got married, and she's been married three times, in order to be more celibate. She said that with all three, after a while, there has been celibacy. It seems that between these marriages she had a lot of affairs.

I have not made a conscious decision. My daughter says I'm on and off celibate, like most people. She's made a decision to be celibate for the moment and I think that it is a relief for her; prior to that she played the field.

I've had more sex since menopause and I've related to men more strongly, but they have been young men. A man of my own age who I met and talked to at a party knocked at the door the other day and I wouldn't let him in the house. I felt, 'Oh has he left his wife, was he having problems in his marriage?' or something like that. I wouldn't think that with a younger man, they have a vitality about them. And with a younger man it's not something that is going anywhere. It's an indulgence that is not permanent.

In my thirties and forties, I didn't notice men at all, I went into sexual purdah for a very long time. If you're damaged by divorce, it can take you years to get over it. I do think there has been some change in me and I feel that a lot of women in their fifties do get this desire. I don't think, 'I want to go to bed with you', that phrase doesn't go through my head, but I am very attracted. I am much more open than I would have been. I talk to men now in a very open way and therefore they feel very relaxed.

I never make the first move, I just don't. I never have, that's why it's so difficult at the moment. Giving out signals is a new thing since menopause, the raging hormones! I'm quite choosy, but there were a couple of men at the party the other night that I thought were quite edible! It's also because I am unshockable, completely unshockable.

I wouldn't have moral objections to sleeping with someone who was married. I was once in love with a friend's husband and once they separated I did have a short affair with him but I have never done it wittingly. You can get very close to somebody's husband, simply because he is the husband of a good friend of yours. I've a couple of friends whose husbands I'm very close to, it's a very relaxing feeling. I've never been put to the test with them.

I always feel reassured that my friends in their late sixties still fancy men and want sex. I don't have a final date in my head. I don't think I will stop fancying men. I don't see myself getting a partner either, I don't think that is in my script at all. I have refused several men recently, it's cheering and slightly bewildering. Sleeping with people can bring back quite painful memories of other relationships if you have been celibate for a long while. An encounter can remind you of a relationship.

I had an encounter with a man in his late forties. Then I slept with him recently. He rang me up and said, 'This is my revenge' because he said I seduced him. He was in my bed anyway, this sounds so barmy! There were lots of people staying and he said, if I have another drink I'll have to stay the night and I said that was fine. Then someone else turned up and all the spare beds were occupied, so I said 'Go and sleep in my bed'. He went to bed, I carried on talking and forgot he was there! I got into bed and the rest is history. Anyway, he rang and said, 'I want you to come over and stay the night'. I said, 'You can't just ask that boldly'. I put the phone down and thought about it and then I suddenly thought, 'Why am I being such a wimp?' So I went upstairs had a bath, took a cab and went over there!

We went to bed and the odd thing is that I have not seen him since. I felt serious scorn for him, there was a built-in rejection there. That decision – getting a cab over to his place – that it was my choice, did make me feel powerful, he was challenging me and that's why I went over there. But it makes me powerful to refuse. Afterwards, I felt a bit of a fool, not like a tart, though, that is an old-fashioned word. It was like the bitter bit really.

I have been less celibate from forty-nine onwards than I have been in prior years. I have slept with more men, but that doesn't mean I have had extended relationships. Five or six. Having sex again did come as a bit of shock, the first two followed one another closely. It was very reassuring but also frightening, because it confirms your solitude, but also you open up by having relationships. It bewildered me, but made me feel fantastic at the same time and then made me feel that I was following the pattern of everybody else. It also saddened me.

I had an affair with a Peruvian, he came on to me. That again was a bit of a shock, I'd had another short affair and I was using one to rub out the other. He was such an exotic creature, with the extraordinary beautiful look that Peruvians have. I was talking to a group of people and he came back to the house and that was a total shock. That was the most frightening thing of all, 'My God where do I go from here?' Luckily I came back to England and got back to normal. It wasn't a holiday romance number at all though.

When I went to bed with the Peruvian, I remember thinking 'This will be something I can tell the grand-children!' It wasn't fun particularly, it was just very good sex! Next day I bolted out of the house and stayed out of the house all day, because it was very much out of character for me to do that. It frightened me, it was like going into unknown territory. I was shocked with myself.

I would never have fallen in love with him, but I could have become quite obsessed with him, and it wouldn't have been reciprocal. I'm too pragmatic, I don't have that much confidence in myself.

I've never slept with a man older than myself in my whole life, ever. I don't think I've slept with more than three middle-aged men in my whole life. I have slept with a forty-six year old recently, who is more of a friend really. During this menopausal crisis, most of the men I have slept with have been between twenty-five and thirty-five. It's been good sexually, very shattering. These are not one-night stands, it's not meet them in the street, go to bed with them and not see them again! With all the men, it worked for me sexually, and all of them have contacted me again, several times.

Younger men are quite intrigued by the idea of older women – not as a permanent fixture, but it's a stage they go through. I don't come on to men, I might talk to them earnestly, that's the closest I ever get, it's a little bit of a teasing thing.

I went to bed with a young man in Poland and he asked me what it felt like to be going to bed with a younger man. I said he was the oldest I had slept with for years, he was thirty-one. He was absolutely furious!

Sally's new-found sexual appetite at menopause marks a liberation in her life that she describes as shocking. She was traumatised by her divorce in the seventies and having to bring up her children single-handed. Like many women left to bring up children, she went into mother mode, and western mother is not sexual. Try walking down the street with a pushchair and see how many admiring glances you get from men. Mother gives strong 'do not touch' signals, a perfect hiding place for someone still getting over a painful separation. Because her children stayed attached to her longer than perhaps is usual, for various complicated reasons, her sexuality was put on hold.

Menopause jerked her back into her own identity as a sexual woman, a physical transformation that has literally shocked her. It's as though she is making up for lost time. Sleeping with much younger men is safe, of course, because she doesn't see them as relationship material. She speaks of her new-found sexual zest with surprise and pleasure, and acknowledges that the next step would be the scary one – having a sexual relationship with someone who might want something more long term.

Maud

Seventy-eight. She was widowed after a long, happy marriage. She dresses fashionably and is conscious of her attraction, but wary of getting involved in other relationships.

I don't have any problem with being celibate, if you want the truth, I masturbate because I feel it's healthy. Sometimes, although I wouldn't dream of getting married because I don't need a man really, I would love one for holidays and going out to dinner. I don't want one bumbling round my flat and I don't think I need him for sex anymore.

I'd be worried about my age – I don't think I want toyboys, I should be worried that they were laughing at me if I were much older. I would be open to another relationship – someone of the same age. If it happened I wouldn't object in any way to the sex, but I would want independence in my home.

If one can achieve orgasm by masturbating, I don't think you want anything else – that sounds rather hard I suppose. I don't want to be cooking another man's meals, I don't want him around all the time, I just want him around when I feel like it.

When I became a widow, men changed a bit, but not as much as I expected. I was quite typical of the emancipated, not-badly-off widow, I was just sixty. No one bothered me, it didn't happen to me at all, in fact probably not as much as I would have liked it to have done!

After he died, it was a great shock, although I was beginning to get a little bit claustrophobic. I liked adventures and travel so almost immediately after he died, I started going off on all sorts of journeys. I went on a freighter to South Africa, to America and all sorts of trips, I went all over the place. I did have a companion but practically hardly anything happened.

He was somebody I used to call my little fat friend – he wasn't very attractive! People who have been attracted to me have always been small men and I can't bear small, fat men. But he was very useful. We met through a friend who thought they would like to do a bit of matchmaking at a dinner party.

He obviously was looking for a companion, so we started going all over the place; we motored down to the south of France. The only thing was he was very mean, I almost always had to pay for myself wherever we went. In a way that gave me the independence I wanted, but also he was very keen on his stomach, he loved his food and that annoyed me because I don't like food all that much. There we were, out in the West Indies, and all he wanted to do was go to a restaurant! I do hear from him still, he is now just eighty. But we've lost touch. We hardly had a physical relationship, there was one occasion when we did go to bed together, but it was such an awful palaver and nothing really happened anyway. I think he was almost incapable anyway at the time. I had had something to drink and I wouldn't have minded.

Since then I have had a relationship with a man I was working with. I got tremendously fond of him, never anything physical, I don't think I ever could have done – the poor man suffered from BO! I really think I was almost in love with him because I loved the work we did together.

One day I went away and when I came back, someone said, 'Have you heard about George, he's died'. I was prepared for my husband to die, but this was a terrible shock. This was about four years ago. Since then I have somebody who is rather fond of me, I think, but he is married. I know the wife and I am very fond of her, I'm not really fond of him, it is just very flattering that's all. So I keep well clear of that!

With women living longer than their husbands, the death of a partner is something many women will have to face in later life. The widow may face a long period of celibacy as she works through the period of grief, after what may be decades of marriage. Many women described the death of a spouse as feeling like they had lost a limb, just getting used to not waking up next to someone seemed impossible at first. Many grief counsellors suggest that it may take several years for the initial period of grief to be worked through, and during that time, the widow gradually gets used to the enforced celibacy. She may find, as Maud has done, that although she still enjoys the company of men, she is reluctant to enter into a new relationship. Maud has found that masturbation fulfils her sexual needs for the moment. When a woman has begun to work through the grief for her husband, why should she automatically want to take on another man? It may be the first time in her life as an adult that she is free to do just as she pleases.

Chapter Six

Self-image

Look in the mirror. Not just a quick glance to make sure your lipstick is on right, but a long, long look. Try five minutes. Do you like what you see? Do you think what nice eyes and lovely skin? Or do you focus on the bits you don't like about yourself? Don't give up, take the full five minutes; do you come up smiling or ready to check into the mother of all liposuction clinics?

This chapter looks at how menopause affects self-image. Television and the media put across clear stereotypes of the post-menopausal woman; she's either a forgetful fool straight out of a sit com, or a dowdy crone. I couldn't think of a single, positive example from television, apart from Miss Marple, but she is an observer, the classic role for powerful older women.

Soaps are particularly at fault. Look at the cast of *EastEnders*, *Brookside* or *Coronation Street*; the older women are all sour-tempered individuals who annoy everyone else. Did menopausal women feel like that? Did they still take care of themselves, look in the mirror, and wear make-up? Were they still worried about body shape, did they diet and feel bad about themselves, or had they finally given up worrying? What about fashion? Was it easy to find attractive clothes? How did others around them react to their menopause? Did they like conforming to the image they saw in the media or did they take pleasure in subverting it?

Self-image is like taking the temperature of the psyche. It can vary from day to day, depending on life events, compliments, hormones or just chance. We all have days when we feel we have nothing to wear, although we have a cupboard full of clothes. Yet on other days, those same clothes make us feel stunning. It's our self-image that makes us feel different.

We learn how to feel about ourselves in early childhood. Were we wanted children? Did our parents give us love and affection and let us know we were great human beings, capable of doing whatever we wanted? What sort of responses did we get from the rest of the family and school? Were there particular circumstances in the family, like illness or abuse, which affected the way we felt about ourselves?

That early external picture we are given of ourselves by others imprints deep patterns. It's a self-fulfilling prophecy; tell a child often enough that they are clumsy and they will begin to drop things. That picture of ourselves is carried into adulthood and reinforced by our experiences of life. It affects the sort of clothes we wear, the partners we choose, how we bring up our own children.

If we have problems with self-image, the longer we leave them untouched, the more difficult they are to heal. The obvious is the physical; most women have bits of themselves that they don't like, but that complete strangers most likely wouldn't notice. You think your elbows stick out, but do you see people peering at them in the street?

For the older woman, menopause may be a time when self-image takes a battering. Some women described how they felt their bodies were beginning to sag and wrinkle, that gravity was beginning to take its toll. But reactions were very different. Some women fought against it, using every device at their disposal, others accepted it was a losing battle, still others welcomed the rest from the fight to appear younger. For certain post-menopausal women, the most important thing was not appearing one's age. The younger the women, the more this was true. Women in their seventies and eighties had mostly acknowledged their age while women in their fifties were still delighted to be mistaken for younger women. In fact, of the much older women, in their seventies and eighties, those who looked physically younger had generally taken good care of themselves, but not become obsessed with their appearance. Women who had been very pretty felt aging to be a welcome relief from all the attention – they could finally be themselves, rather than the person this pretty little thing was supposed to be.

Older women still thought it important to take care of themselves, but it was often on their own terms; they no longer had to dress for success or seduction, they could dress as they pleased, sometimes for the first time in their lives.

But can aging be separated from the menopause? Because it happens to a woman in her fifties, menopause is often taken as an unwelcome sign of impending mortality, some women talked about the panic at the thought of death that menopause brought on. But menopause is surely just a step in the aging process, like any other milestone. I was struck time and time again during these interviews by the difficulty of putting an age on any of these women. Some I would have put fifteen years younger than their age, others appeared older, but I don't think I could have guessed one correctly. They were the age they felt in their heads, whether they are the seventy year old still disco dancing or the woman in her fifties not daring to wear trendy clothes until she had tried wearing them in the house!

The idea of not looking one's age is constantly reinforced by advertising. Advertisements in women's magazines have recently adopted a quasi-scientific language to
make us buy small pots of extremely expensive lotions and
potions. What we are buying is magic, an offering to the
goddess of youth – the more expensive the pot, the more
we believe in its properties.

Low self-image stopped women from enjoying life.
Some women spoke of debilitating depression and a
lifetime of anxiety and tranquillisers. The older women
with depression tended to try and cope on their own,
although one woman in her seventies had gone to therapy
to sort herself out. The younger the women were, the more
likely they were to consult experts or try and get help from
an outside agency.

Low self-image seems to be directly linked to difficulty
with menopause. Every single woman who had serious
problems with menopause had suffered from low self-
image and depression beforehand. If women feel bad
about themselves, the physical symptoms of menopause
can make them plunge further into depression. But
menopause can also be a baptism of fire; many women
felt that they had been waiting all their lives to come to
terms with their problems, and that menopause finally
gave them the excuse to deal with feelings of low self-
worth. Other people expect women to behave strangely
during menopause, it's the perfect time to bring out all the
suitcases of rubbish they have been dragging behind them
all their lives, open them up, and finally rummage around
in there.

Marjorie

*Seventy-six. She is dressed in a black leather trouser suit which she
adores because it's stylish and with the dogs, she doesn't have to
brush herself down before she goes out of the house. She has recently*

had an eye operation and apologises for looking a fright, which she doesn't at all. She's carefully made up and draws admiring glances when she walks me through town back to the station.

Why shouldn't I be smart? I've never dressed like the little old ladies in the high street. I've always dressed adapting the style of the times. Because at this age I've been through the thirties, the forties, the fifties, the sixties and now God help up us, we're in the nineties. I'm not so much interested in fashion as style. I have my own style and I stick to it. I'm not, and I never have been, miniskirt material, I'm too long in the leg and too short in the body. I know myself pretty well by now. I'm not mutton dressed as lamb, I hope.

Some older women think they have no right to be smart, people tell them that and they believe it, but I get very cross with some people, the way they don't take any interest in themselves. They stop taking an interest and cut off at menopause, as if it's somehow sinful to be interested in anything else. You might as well say that you mustn't be interested in books or food or the cinema! I still wear make-up, it modifies itself through the years, obviously.

I'm not pleased with the way I look, I was ugly to start with, and I'll be ugly to finish with. One does the best with what God has given you, and one's very grateful, because there are so many people who are so much worse off. There are lots of bits of me that I am not happy with. I'd still have a nose job if I could afford it, except that I've got better ways of spending the money now. As you get older, you say, 'I can't do anything about it, so I had better just push on with it, do the best I can'. Maximise the positive and minimise the negative.

I still go out whenever I can. I'm not going to be stuck in here just because they say that it's dangerous out there. I go on group activities, I'm not a bit worried about going to things by myself. I never have been. I love any sort of gig or dancing. I can gyrate gently, I love music, so I always have a good time.

Marjorie challenges many people's view of what older women should look like and how they should behave. Disco dancing at seventy-six seems bizarre at first, but why should it? Is there a cut off point for having fun?

Marjorie has been active in local environmental politics and I can see the tabloid headlines now – 'Groovy granny goes green'. But the tabloid mentality we all carry in our heads, the reduction of individuals to how we think they should behave, needs to be challenged. Its simplistic categorising leaves no room for the individuality of someone as joyful as Marjorie.

Katherine

Fifty-three. We meet at her office and she's smartly and fashionably dressed with much attention to detail. The green of her cashmere jumper exactly matches the green check of her skirt, and is picked out by pink coral beads. She is carefully made up.

I still worry about the way I look, far too much. It's become of concern to me, partly that has to do with the way my husband emphasises my looks. It's almost a matter of pride that I feel I don't look fifty-three. My children have also done that to me. They've said, 'Don't buy that, it makes you look mumsy' – they're proud to have a mother who looks good and still flashes the old legs a bit.

Also there will come a time when things will change and droop, so I might as well make the most of them now! I do like looking attractive. I do feel good about myself on the whole. I could wish for a smaller stomach, that's my fault for drinking gin and tonics. I don't eat that much really, so that doesn't bother me, and I do a lot of walking. I'm really quite healthy considering that I abuse myself from time to time.

You just get used to the bits that you are fed up with, every so often I think, if I really cut down on the gin and tonics and the lager at the weekend and I did some exercising, that stomach would go, but then I think why the hell bother! I've had it this long and it doesn't seem to have hampered me, so why bother. I mean if I got violently fat I would do something about it.

I feel more easy with myself, not so devastated by the fact that I haven't got legs up to my ears, like some people. Obviously there are things I wish I had. I wish I hadn't smoked this long and I wish I'd kept up the exercise a bit more. I used to be a ballet dancer in my teenage years and I've kept pretty good shape after babies and things, but I have let it all go a bit.

I used to be much more worried about the way I looked, much more concerned about clothes and being in style and being a pretty young thing because it was the sixties – image was a lot to do with it and having the right haircut. But actually, when you see the kind of people that attract each other, you can see the physical side isn't that important in the end and you think however I get, it's still going to be OK.

Also there are different people for different people. You can't please everybody, so be happy with what you are. People like all different things. I worked for an agency that had lots of fat people on their books. They had this huge woman on their books, enormous, but the sexiest person you ever met. They did a television programme about her and she got thousands of letters proposing marriage, so there's somebody for everybody!

Katherine gives out conflicting messages about her self-image. She's smartly and fashionably dressed and looks a lot younger than she is. But her self-image is split in two. All the pleasure in her appearance is handed over to others, her husband and her children. She is left with only dissatisfaction about her height, her stomach, her fitness and smoking. She seems to be fighting a losing battle to please others and only others; the pride she takes in her appearance is reflected glory.

Jenny

Fifty-four. She is divorced with three children, two with serious learning difficulties. She has been in therapy to sort out problems with cruelty in childhood and is now dating again, much to her amusement.

I feel I've got something to offer now, whereas I didn't before. Initially, in my first marriage, I exchanged sex for affection. I was very desperate for affection, never having had it at all at home. I equated one with the other. Just to have someone there. My first marriage was pretty disastrous. Certainly I like sex much more than when I was in my twenties. It does surprise me but it's very nice!

It works better as you get older and gain confidence and experience – the confidence that goes with the knowledge. I can talk about sex now with partners and ask for what I like. And if they have inhibitions, you can get round that, and encourage them to talk about sex. I think it's very important to talk about sex and what we both want.

It surprises me how much I've changed since menopause, how much freer I feel. I'm much more emotionally stable and calmer. I don't get worked up about things, I'm more objective about things which means I'm more relaxed. I've got a lot of confidence in me. Ten years ago I was a shadow of what I am now. When I was on the beach on holiday I envied the young girls with their young, lithe bodies. I thought, 'Aren't they lovely, while I'm here getting older all the time'. It's sad that older women don't have such a sexy image, the idea that we are just comfortable.

Am I keener on sex? Difficult to say when you haven't had it for a while! I think I am, though I didn't expect that, it's very surprising somehow. I didn't expect it at all.

I still worry about the way I look and I diet, and changing rooms in shops are the worst, aren't they! I'm still very aware of my shape, because it's so horrendous! I'm going to join a gym with my daughter and tone myself up a bit. I am very aware of what I look like, I like to look nice. I'm quite grey really but I wouldn't let myself be grey. When you'r grey, you think of yourself as much older; it's all tied up with your sexuality, you look like an old woman because you are grey.

You can't prevent yourself from looking older, but you can do quite a lot. Also having a fourteen-year-old daughter who says, 'Mum I would just die if my friends knew you had grey hair'. She's very aware of having an older mum, all her friends' mothers are late thirties.

I've never let myself go, I've always liked to look as reasonable as I can. Men can get away with more, in their fifties and sixties they are on the whole looking at younger women because it boosts their egos, doesn't it, to have a nice-looking woman on their arm.

I don't think discontent diminishes with age, if anything it gets worse. My thighs! If I came back in another life, one thing I would like is to be slimmer. I have great difficulty keeping my weight under control, it's only the fact that I am tall that disguises it.

I'm very much more positive about myself. I don't flirt, I wouldn't know how, I say that with all humility, I wish I could flirt. Some women can really flirt with men, but I can't it's not me. But I can be myself more than I could when I was younger. I take the view that you are what you are, and we're all very different, and not everyone likes everyone else. You can't change what you are, and people must accept you for what you are. I've accepted myself, up to a point. I've done a lot of thinking.

I went to counselling after my marriage broke up, to a male psychologist. I didn't feel he was a lot of help. We talked about the marriage and other problems. He kept on saying I was coping beautifully and I felt he was a bit patronising. The theory was praise the person, and that's not what I wanted, I knew I was a mess, so I didn't go any more.

I left it until two years ago when I was feeling very low. I really doubted myself and my own sexuality, I hit a bad patch. This counsellor was a woman and she was excellent, I felt I could talk to her. I talked about my mother and all those angry feelings, and how she had totally destroyed my self-esteem. We talked about the break-up and relationships, we talked about everything. My self-esteem has returned after a lot of hard work and thinking things over.

Life seems clearer, very much so. It's a result of both menopause and counselling. I'm not looking for the moon any more. I know what I want. Sometimes your expectations can be so high, you'll never achieve them, you have to settle for what you've got. I can see the way ahead in a way I couldn't before, sometimes it looks a bit black, I don't like the thought of retirement. I'm a busy person and the thought of having to slow down isn't a nice thought, but then I think you come to accept things as life goes along. Each stage that you get to, you go along with it and your body slows down. Retirement is the next big hurdle, so the longer I can postpone it the better! Things change, they never stay the same. What's the good of worrying about it, you might as well enjoy things as they are.

Jenny's self-image has never been better than it is now. The damage done to her in childhood has been resolved through therapy, and she has finally been able to drop the heavy weight of low self-esteem that has been dragging her down all her life.

Physically she is like most women – there's a bit of her that she'd like to swap for another version. But Jenny has realised that all women feel like that. Women are encouraged to be unhappy with our bodies, it gives us something to worry about, gets us to buy expensive potions and lotions and stops us getting on with our lives.

Brenda

Fifty-four. She is happily married with a strong sexual relationship. She is fashionably and stylishly dressed although she admits to being nervous about high fashion and wishes trendier clothes were available to older women. She still buys trendy outfits and wears them at home or on holiday first to try them out.

I didn't work all the first years of my married life. I enjoyed it. I wouldn't admit this to many people but I loved being a mum! I felt it was challenging me. On my CV, I put family management, I'm really quite proud. I like everything about being at home. I did part-time bits like Avon and I never worried about money; not that it wasn't an issue, I always felt that I was making a really good contribution, I knew what money was coming in.

But when I was forty my husband was made redundant, he couldn't get a job and one of us had to do something about it, so I had to go back to work! It wasn't my choice then, I had a lovely clique of friends and I was quite happy. I got a management post in a public relations firm. I managed nineteen staff. Then about three years ago I was made redundant. I was conscious then that no one wants you when you're fifty, a woman and if they think you're technical.

My husband's working again now, but I haven't been tempted to give up work – for a person who's been made redundant, who says she loves being at home, that seems incredible! I took another job, I've been working here three years now, but I don't really like it. When I was made redundant, I wanted to be a counsellor. Nobody told me it was bloody hard work to be a counsellor!

I applied for a counselling skills and attitudes course, but in the meantime I got a job here on a six-month contract. I had problems deciding, but they gave me half a day off to do this course for two years. That's kept me going to be honest. Years ago, I read a magazine that talked all about counselling and I knew that was what I wanted to do. But I was in such a good job, bringing in more money than my husband, I got a company car, mobile telephone and I couldn't give that up to do something I really wanted, so I kept on in that job. When I was made redundant, I thought 'Now I can do something that I really want to do'. I was toying with regret, living to a lifestyle with my money, and could I give all that up to do something that I really wanted to do? I couldn't, I felt terribly selfish.

I feel I'm in a different place than I was four years ago, emotionally I have to be very aware. I'm quite a confident person, but when I was made redundant and then coming to this job, which is quite menial, it rocked my confidence completely.

I still worry about the way I look, that doesn't change! I think the fact that I'm putting on weight and having to rinse my hair because I'm totally grey now and I hate spending time at the hairdressers on the colour. I try not to, I don't like what I see in the mirror, so I don't dwell on it.

There's a feeling that you just want to stay young. I didn't think I flirted, but friends say that I do. Friends say that I'm naïve because I talk to people and sometimes flirt with them but I wouldn't assume that anyone would fancy me. I know that's daft but I just wouldn't assume that anyone would, so I feel completely free to flirt.

Like many women, Brenda feels guilty at the idea of doing what she really wants to do in life. We have been brought up as women to believe that our lives should be wholly in the service of others. But society is changing; women are now encouraged to lead more fulfilling lives themselves, but still to continue being the emotional providers. So choosing what we want to do ourselves – whether it's being a full-time mum or leaving a well-paid job to follow a different career path – makes us feel guilty.

Rose

Eighty-four. She is a pensioner living in a sheltered council flat on a sunny square. The flat is spotless, she washed the walls down herself last year, she tells me. She is active in older women's rights and shocked by current government attitudes to the elderly. A gentle, strong woman who has always had to struggle financially.

I try to keep up my appearance, I have a very small pension and yet I manage. I go into the charity shops and I buy myself something smart. There are bits of myself that I don't like – me feet! I've got terrible feet, terrible hands, I've had to work so hard, washing and cleaning. I've always kept myself roughly the same weight. I take good care of myself. Don't sit with a long face, put lots of cream on it and smile.

Rose is the embodiment of making the best of things. Her positive attitude to life, in the face of enormous financial and health difficulties, has left her, at eighty-four, with the serenity of a life well lived.

Annie

Fifty-six. She feels unhappy about her appearance, making reference to herself in deprecating terms during the interview. She refers to a problem with food when she opens a newly bought

packet of biscuits, saying. 'I won't have one or I will eat them all'.
She seems at a low ebb. She is cheerful only when talking about the
past and her cats. Therapy has helped her maintain a status quo.
She feels being gay exacerbates her problems; both lowering the
chances of meeting a new partner and fighting the opinions and
prejudices of the straight world.

One factor that has stopped me getting into a relationship, these nine celibate years, is the fact that after my last partner left me, I went into a very bad depression. I had lost my house, lost my way of life. I did have a fleeting relationship with a woman, to whom I absolutely lost my heart, I was on the rebound. I fell desperately in love with her and she seemed to be playing about with me. She found someone else, and then said, 'You didn't think it was going to last did you? You are too old for me.' And then I was attacked in the street by a man. It was a sexual attack, although he didn't manage to do much because I screamed and yelled, but the upshot was that I got myself into therapy. He told me he had a knife and I suddenly realised while he had his arm round my neck, that the first thought that went through my head was, 'If you're going to kill me, I hope you do it quickly, because it will save me the trouble of having to do it myself'.

As soon as I started examining what had gone through my head, I realised how depressed I was and really felt my depression. I got myself into therapy with a wonderful woman therapist and I fell in love with her, of course. It's par for the course, I know, I made the mistake of making her very central to my life.

If all else failed, I would get to her every Friday, she was the person who filled up my thoughts and my dreams. We're not talking a very glamourous woman here, or a very young woman, she was a bit younger than me. I was in therapy with her for eight years, I stopped last year. It took me a whole year to prise myself away from her, during which time I went into the most appalling depression, I still am rather depressed now. That was one of the factors that stopped me finding anyone else. Because while she was in my life, although it's not a proper relationship in that way, not even a social relationship, I just felt that she was enough, while she was there everything was OK.

It is a normal part of therapy, the transference, and had I also been in a relationship with someone else, that transference wouldn't have been so strong. I said to her while I was trying to prise myself away from her, 'I shouldn't have let this happen should I?' She said I couldn't help it, if it hadn't happened we wouldn't have got so far in therapy. Did it help my depression, bearing in the mind that I have been feeling dreadful for about a year, possibly not!

It helped me in other ways. I'm sure I am wiser, I'm much more relaxed, a much less edgy person than I was. I'm still capable of becoming very depressed, I always will be. I have been on the verge of topping myself many times. I think I would, if it weren't for the fact that I wouldn't want to upset my family and friends, and who is going to look after my animals? They have been my lifeline sometimes.

Why should we rush around trying to be sexual all the time? You may notice that I'm not wearing make-up, I haven't worn it for many years, but of course that's not to do with age. We shouldn't be press ganged into feeling that we must be in a relationship, or we must be having sex the whole time. I think that is wrong. But to shut up shop and start shuffling round in black, I really don't want to do that either, there's something nice about feeling sexual.

There are enormous chunks of myself that I don't like, and it gets worse with age. I have in my lifetime been too thin, and I adored it, I loved it. I can still remember the days when I used to squeeze myself into a little pair of tight jeans, a tiny T-shirt and a pair of trainers. I mourn for that self, which is not going to come back again. I only ever lose weight if I'm either having a nervous breakdown or I'm in love. When neither is happening to me, my metabolism slows down.

I stopped smoking, took early retirement from my job two years ago and became menopausal; three things that are guaranteed to make you put on weight. I would feel better in my clothes if I was thinner. I'm on tenterhooks these days, thinking 'I hope to God no one asks me out anywhere smart, because I haven't got any clothes'.

I can't fit into them, and if I went out to get something I would still look like shit, like half the side of a barrage balloon, so what's the point? I hate seeing myself in a mirror or a shop window. You will notice that this is a flat full of all sorts of things, but not full of mirrors. There's one in the bathroom from the neck up! I've always had a very bad body image. I'd like to be thin, if I were thin, I'd feel sexier. I always feel younger and better looking when I'm thin, my face gets thinner. I don't look so much like my mum, I look more like my dad which is important to me.

I thought to myself the other day, 'If I don't look to having a sexual relationship anymore, why the hell am I worried about what I look like?' But I suppose at the same time I don't feel ready to wear baggy old clothes and really go down hill, there's a tiny little smidgeon that hasn't given up!

The fact that Annie couldn't look at herself full length even if she wanted to, because she has no mirrors in her flat, underlines how low her self-image is. She mourns for her thin self, knows that person will never return, yet has put her life on hold in the meantime. Her self-image stops her buying new clothes and accepting social invitations. This leads to a vicious circle of comfort eating – those choccy biscuits – which leaves her feeling

worse about herself. To break the cycle, she has to come to terms
with the here and now, not the what if scenario.

Elizabeth

Seventy-seven. She is married to a man who can't show affection to
anybody, so she lavishes affection on her children and grand-
children. She had two of her children in her forties. Her husband
is now disabled and becoming more dependent and even more
resentful of her. She seems to be making some tough decisions
about the future and feels a new kind of strength emerging.

I don't pamper myself, I don't go in for lots of creams and
lotions, I just put a bit of moisturising cream on and a bit
of cover-up stuff, a little bit of eye shadow and mascara.
My skin is getting very dry, that is age of course, also I'm
on these water reducing tablets. I'm interested in clothes
but not obsessively so, and, of course, really until the last
few years I've never had much to spend on dress. When
the children were smaller, I used to call myself second-
hand Rose, because everything I had was second hand! I
do still pop into the hospice shops and if there's something
nice, I have it. I can't really remember when I last went
into a shop and bought an outfit – oh, yes when my
youngest son got married, that's about seven years ago! I
get things through catalogues.

I've become much more tolerant, I'm more fulfilled
now. I've allowed myself to have more interests. I do a lot
of reading, I listen to music that *I* like whereas before I
wouldn't have done. Fortunately with the advent of
Classic FM even my husband has begun to like classical
music. Before, although I had classical records, I never
put them on when he was around, he wasn't that interested in music, whereas it has always been terribly
important to me.

I have begun to realise that my wants and desires are as

important as his. This has come very late, very late indeed. I was quite shocked when I went out shopping with my daughter and said casually that I didn't buy certain things because James didn't like them. 'Oh,' she said, 'I don't buy what I don't like!' That's the modern attitude, it's quite different.

Also the realisation that basically he is a very selfish man. I did have confidence when I was younger but you lose your confidence terribly quickly when you stop working. It's quite awful how women do lose confidence in themselves when they are home all day, coping with the children. It is an extremely demanding job, running the home and making the money go as far as it should go, but they still lose their confidence. It's not valued at all.

Now I'm having to take on more responsibility with his disability, and he is hating every minute of it. I try not to let it be too obvious, because I know how he hates it, he insists on keeping control. He's always kept the most meticulous accounts, but now I have to do them. But he sits beside me and makes sure that I'm doing it just as he wants it done. It drives me mad, he queries everything. He always has queried everything, he'll never accept anything at its face value. There are occasions when I just have to walk out and go for a walk down the road otherwise I would scream blue murder.

I've got to the age when I would like to shrug off the responsibility, I'd love to be just taken care of. I do get desperately tired now, and it is then that I think, 'Oh dear, if someone would just look after me, because I have been looking after people all my life'.

Elizabeth's daughter highlights the difference between the generations. While Elizabeth still tries to be generous and considerate to a man who never seems to have had a thought for anyone else, her daughter puts her own needs on an equal footing with those of her husband.

The problem with giving your life entirely to others and not saving time and space for yourself is that there is no end to it, as Elizabeth is beginning to realise. She has taken on the role of always being there, providing and comforting, and at seventy-seven she would like some comfort herself. But part of the problem is that she is not used to seeing her needs met and doesn't know how to begin to ask.

I wonder, on the way home, if her husband has ever worn second-hand clothes, somehow I doubt it.

Judith

Sixty-two. She is widowed. She giggles a lot during our interview and has a good sense of humour. She has recently returned to work part time after retirement, this has done her ego good – she says that they can't quite manage without her still. She has taken care over her appearance and is carefully made up. She has a beautiful, newly decorated home in a small village in the country.

I'm not 100 per cent happy with the way I look, there are definitely bits I'd like to change [*she laughs*]. I wish my legs were a bit longer and a bit slimmer I suppose. I wish that my tummy was a bit flatter, like it used to be. I wish I were prettier, more beautiful.

One of my main worries is my hair, I do like my hair to look nice. I am pretty conscious of self-image and I want to try and keep reasonably in shape, I do dread looking old and frumpy, definitely.

You do come to accept your body as you get older. I've been in it a long time now, so I know it pretty well and I know what suits me and I suppose really, on the whole, I know how to make the best of it, when I want to. My body was better when I was younger, when I was twenty, obviously, but that wouldn't suit me now at the age I am. I'm more content than I was twenty years ago. I never felt I was perfect, I always wished something was a bit different. I accept it now, and think, 'Well you're stuck with it and you're not going to change it', so I don't try too hard.

I don't diet, not desperately so. Sometimes I think, 'Oh gosh you've filled out round the tummy, you must go easy on the sweet things for a bit'; then I will half-heartedly diet for a while, but not seriously, because I'm much too fond of food! I exercise in moderation, I have spasms when I think, I'll jog round the block each day, I'll go the gym and lay on the floor and do tummy exercises, and I will for a few days, but it passes off fairly quickly usually!

You can be the person you want to be at my age. The quest for a mate and a family is much less urgent, in fact it has almost disappeared, so I tend to please myself more, do what I like doing more, dress the way I want to, more than I might have. I'm not the slavish follower of fashion I was in my younger days, because fashion one thinks, attracts the opposite sex. You have to wear the clothes all the other girls are wearing or you will miss out because you won't be as attractive. I used to go to dances because it was the place to be, that's where you met the boys, whereas now, one of the last places I would want to go to is a dance, where again one might meet possible partners. That just doesn't appeal to me particularly. It's a relief in a way to be able to say, 'If I don't like doing that, I won't'.

Judith knows and likes her body; it's like a favourite jumper, a little worn at the seams, but comfortable and reassuring. So what makes Judith's attitude so different from Katherine's or Annie's? Liking yourself is to do with acceptance – not resignation but a recognition of good and bad points, changing the bits that can be improved and coming to terms with the rest. However, Judith still suffers from Sunday supplement syndrome. We all read those articles when people describe their day and by eight o'clock, they've run five miles, showered and breakfasted, caught up with their correspondence and read three chapters of War and Peace.

Clare

Fifty-six. She is living with a husband in bad health. She is slim and fashionably dressed, and she works part time in a charity shop.

I do take good care of myself, I like to look nice. My image is important to me, you read articles about women who reach middle age not caring about themselves, slopping around in whatever. With two daughters who like looking nice as well, that helps. Going to work is another thing keeping me looking reasonable. I do some yoga, I like to try and keep fit. There are bits of myself I don't like, certainly as you get older you seem to thicken! Recently I had a birthday and Stephen said he would buy me some clothes. Everything I put on I thought I looked awful in, so I stomped out of the shop!

I haven't come to terms with myself yet. I'm a very introverted person, very shy, timid, although perhaps meeting people the first time, I don't give that impression. I haven't got a very high esteem of myself, and that is connected with our problems. When we married he was a vicar; one thinks the stereotypical vicar and family, but it wasn't like that. To start with we were very hard up, then he had to leave the job here because of his drinking. It was in the local paper and it was pretty traumatic, for a long time I felt that if I was in the village, people would point me out.

But then Stephen was happy working abroad, he is an extremely good vicar. He's good at looking after others, hopeless at looking after himself. He's a very thoughtful, very kind person. Young people love going to him because he listens well, and he gets on well with elderly people. He doesn't ever have time to think of himself, he thinks it wrong to think of himself.

I did have a good model from my parents. I knew they had a good sexual relationship from the way they were together, from the things my mother said, hints that she dropped. My mother died at sixty-nine, he did meet someone else, they didn't ever get married but he was seventy-four. My father was a lovely man, very attracted to ladies and basically he was desperately lonely. Although he was very faithful to my mother, he couldn't bear being without a lady.

It was rather admirable because he was very shy. I really took my hat off to him, he put his name down in one of these agencies. They didn't ever marry or move in together, she'd come and stay with him. I thought it was great, I was very pleased. He died when he was ninety, and it continued until the last couple of years. He had a stroke and she was getting a bit senile and couldn't understand, but she would still go and visit him, and they would always hold hands and have a cuddle. He gave me a good image of myself. He used to compliment us on outfits that we wore or if he liked our hair.

When Clare married a vicar, one of the copers in the community, she discovered that they can't always deal with their own problems. The positive self-image she got from her parents, particularly her father, has been dented by her inability to get through to her husband. Their sexual problems have been compounded by lack of communication, until a vicious circle has been set up. Low self-image can be highly infectious, it seems Clare has caught a bad dose of it from her husband.

Caroline

Seventy-three. She has had much to cope with in life. A brother died in childhood of meningitis, and another brother was stillborn after her mother was hit in the abdomen with a cricket ball. As the only surviving child, she had to learn to cope with her parents' protectiveness. She has married three times, firstly to a man who ran off with someone else, then to a concentration camp survivor who died, and finally to her first husband again. Her grown-up children continue to be a cause for concern; she is very much the coper in the family.

I've always been very strong, perhaps too strong! I've always been very healthy, never had any illnesses – I was brought up in the country. My mother was a strong character, so I had a good model in her. People needing emotional help have always appealed to me, it's something to do with my brother's illness, I developed a caring side.

I feel I'm quite strong, I've had to weather quite a few storms in my life; I've had to make big decisions by myself. Physically I suppose you get used to yourself. I suppose we'd all like to be slimmer and more elegant, those sort of things, but it doesn't bother me, there's nothing major.

Caroline's self-image pattern was laid down in childhood when the family went through such tragedy. Not only did she become the focus of all her parents' love, but all their anxiety as well. It sounds like she had to parent her own parents through their grief, and she learnt to be a coper from an early age. When her first marriage failed, she married a concentration camp survivor, someone else who desperately needed her. The danger of love as social work is that you don't have time for your own needs.

Madeleine

Seventy-three. She has a very happy marriage. She is aware that the physical changes brought on by age can have unexpected benefits.

I was pretty when I was young and I took the attention as my due, I enjoyed it! I don't think I was bigheaded about it, I just knew people were nice to me. I would flirt up to a point, but not if they got too near. If you are pretty, you have a difficult relationship with the world because people judge you, even though you don't want them to. That's the sad thing, all these lovely girls who don't look like Cindy Crawford are being overlooked, and yet they would be far more satisfying as partners.

I was liked and I didn't have to work at it, it was just there. I never had to get through a barrier and prove myself in any way, men always came to me, which I realise is very unfair, but it helps in relationships.

People did take me seriously at work though, because they do if you know your work. In fact I used to hope to get to a point where they didn't see you as a woman, they saw you for what you were producing.

All that prettiness has gone. I'm a gran now, part of the older generation. Now I'm all sagged and bagged. There are bits I don't like, the cheeks are all going. Is it worth going to have a tuck? No, I can't be bothered. I was always eight and half stone, now I am up to nine stone, so I feel if it creeps on, I'll do something about it. I've always been used to being active and lithe. I'm friends with my body, pretty well, and thank God it hasn't let me down and I don't have any illnesses. It's done me well. I don't worry about my appearance, I've dressed up for you today, but I'm usually so casual I'm verging on the scruffy! I feel thankful to my body, I live in it and it doesn't cause me a lot of trouble.

Like Judith, Madeleine feels comfortable with herself and is grateful for her good health. The double bind of beauty, that people are attracted to you but don't take you seriously, fades with the years. We are all drawn by good looks and make assumptions about character from them. The super models make the standard impossible, they are beautiful freaks of nature. For the rest of us to aspire to those looks is to set ourselves up to fail. Their whole raison d'être is to look different from the rest of us, hence the media and fashion houses are always desperately searching for the new look, the new face that can express our longing for perfection.

Mavis

Seventy-three. She was widowed after a happy second marriage. A bundle of energy and fun, she takes great care over her appearance and thinks younger generations don't care enough what they look like. Recently she had an affair with a forty-four year old man she describes as delightful. She is close to her family.

Other people can't understand how I've kept so young. I suppose I've always had a good sex life! That's the secret, not that I've got one now. I have always felt that if I've been having a good sexual relationship, then I have felt better. It is good for you, it always made me feel very, very well.

So many people get to a certain age, maybe forty or fifty and they feel that's it, they're old. You don't have to age, just carry on day after day, month after month, and take life as it comes. What's the point of putting up with it and not enjoying it? It's what makes me feel good, happy, relaxed and fit. I look at myself and think, 'Well, you're not doing so bad and sex has got something to do with it'.

Many women of my generation have missed out, a lot of women even now think sex is a dirty word, you mustn't enjoy it. Sex is to have children, not let's turn the cooker off and go to bed for an hour! That's what it's all about.

When you're getting older, your skin is very, very important. I wouldn't dream of walking out of the house without any make-up on or not having my hair done! I still look in the mirror – a lot of women give up, I don't know why. There are times when I go to the bathroom and think, 'I've been doing this for years and years, why I am still doing it', but I still do it. I do it for myself.

Discontent does diminish with age. I think it's acceptance, you reach a stage, I've hit my head on this so many times, I do have to accept the way I am. It's you.

Sex as a panacea for aging? Mavis may have come up with the buzz idea of the nineties, after aerobics and the high-fibre diet. She reckons that it doesn't matter if you're not having sex now, as long as you had good sex at some time in your life, rather like saving for a rainy day. If it makes you look as good as she does, there may be something in the theory. Mavis was recently approached in the street by a dating agency who wanted to put her on their books. She was flattered and they were astonished when she told them her age.

Sally

Fifty two. After a life of looking after children as a single parent, menopause seems to have liberated her sexuality. She's particularly attracted by younger men and they certainly respond.

I don't know what it is about menopause that has made me more sexual. I'm not as attractive as I was ten years ago, no doubt about it. Ten years ago I felt bloody fed up, but I looked great and didn't know it. I'm less self-conscious, less burdened, more vital perhaps and men are responding to that.

My self-image is not very good at the moment, I feel I have to take steps about the way I look. I'm not committed, I'm delaying it. This morning I went out of the house very fast and I met two people and I loathe the fact that I met them looking dishevelled! I wish, like my mother did, that I'd put my make-up on before I had opened the front door.

When I look at myself in the mirror, I see somebody who needs to lose weight. My teeth gave me a lot of problems recently, but are now sorted out. The teeth thing is a joke with my friends, we are all losing our teeth or they are cracking. It's worse if I catch glances of myself in photographs – mirrors are very good really because you lift your head up and you don't see yourself in profile.

Most women that I know and like a lot are not hugely

thin. The balance has tipped, I'm much more interested in fitness now.

I'm less discontented – my self-image has always been bad, but I worry about it less now. When I think, 'God, you look awful', I don't think I'm going to cut my throat, I just accept it. I haven't become comfortable in my body, definitely not, absolutely not. But I've given up wildly serious, extreme dieting.

Sally is getting positive reinforcement about her self-image from all the younger men who are chasing her since she came into her own at menopause. She acknowledges, ruefully, that her body is changing, her weight distribution is different, her teeth are suffering. But menopause has also taught her to seize the day, she realises that she was in better shape ten years ago, but was too depressed to take advantage of it. Now something has shifted and she has come to an acceptance of herself which makes her attractive to others.

Mary

Forty-seven. She had an accelerated menopause after a hysterectomy which led to severe depression and an exaggeration of all the classic menopausal symptoms.

When I was severely depressed my self-image was a problem. I still showered everyday, sometimes I couldn't be bothered with my hair, I'd just put it up in a bun or tie it back for speed. I'd just sling any dress on, but deep down I knew that I hadn't bothered as much as I would have liked to. I like the way I look now, I've got quite a good self-image. Before the hysterectomy it wasn't so good, I was working so hard, it was a case of shower, get dressed and slap my make-up on. I still did bother, but I found it an effort because I was on the go all the time.

I hate my stomach, always have done since I had my children. It's funny really because nobody else notices.

I've generally liked the way I looked, I've always been very critical if something's not right, I'm not happy until I have put it right.

Mary seems to have spent much of her life too busy to have time to bother with herself. Self-worth can slip away if it is not regularly maintained. It's a bit like servicing the car, you think it's all right, until it breaks down in the middle of nowhere in the pouring rain. Mary focused her dissatisfaction on her stomach, but she admits that no one else notices it. Many women have a favourite part of themselves they love to hate. It's a convenient scapegoat for all that is not right in their lives.

Maud

Seventy-eight. She is widowed, and a strong minded, confident woman who has taken great care over her appearance.

I try and look after myself. I still use make-up and I still like clothes but I feel that is a question of self-respect as much as anything. I don't do it consciously to attract anybody, it's important to me, myself. Older women can begin to get quite disgusting and I just hope that I won't get to that point. I still look in the mirror and worry, I do mind about the way I look. Everybody has bits they don't like, it must increase with age. I do envy the young when they look so beautiful, I'm amazed how beautiful everyone is today.

I get lonely, in a very deep down way, but I'm very busy all the time. I feel I'm a bit on a roundabout and don't want to get off. I daren't get off, I shall just disintegrate into old age if I do. I'm beginning to shed some things, but I still like doing lots of things.

Is Maud right to cling on to activities and remain as busy and occupied as possible? The alternative is to vegetate, if you don't use it, you lose it. Many older women seem to age suddenly, it's as if time has caught up with them. Keeping busy and active really does seem to mean that you stay as old as you feel. Travel, exercise, theatre and cinema all encourage us to remain a part of the world, rather than disengaging into the slow spiral to death.

Dot

Seventy. She feels she has come into her own since menopause. She is now relaxed with herself, comfortable in her clothes and body.

I've got so much more since I retired. I've got over the person I was then, who was always afraid that something might go wrong. I counsel people of my own age, and you only have to listen to your dreams and listen to how much is still there. People can change at any time in their lives, that's really important, it's a slow process but you can get there.

I care about what I want to wear now, instead of what other people want me to wear. I used to dress exactly as I ought to dress, and I absolutely loathed it, so now people will take me as I am. That means that I like to keep reasonably trim, I feel ugly if I am too large so I am careful and I do take exercise, that is very important, I try to encourage other people to do so too.

I wish I hadn't given my face quite so much sun, so that it wasn't quite so wrinkled. It's a terrific temptation to have it done, purely because then I know I would really get away with it. My daughter and my granddaughter say don't, because they want it to be the face that has been lived in. At times I'm proud of that, other times I look in the mirror without my glasses on and it's fine, and then I put my glasses on and say, 'Oh God no!'

I'm very fortunate, although I don't like the lines, there's not much else I don't like about myself. I'd love to have had lovely hair, lots of it. It's always been a burden, I'm lucky that I haven't gone grey, we don't in my family.

My discontent has diminished with age but I'm sure that that is not generally true. I think for 90 per cent of people, it's hell getting older. I am one of the very fortunate ones who feel that I escape more and more into greater happiness, greater awareness and spirituality. I feel that if I can come to the time of my death knowing that it means absolutely nothing to me, then I will be thrilled to bits, because I believe that is where we all ought to be.

Dot is exceptional, her self-image has never been better. But after a lifetime of tranquillisers and anxiety, it could hardly have got worse. Menopause has given her new vitality and self-worth, a chance to explore new avenues of counselling and spirituality. To lift or not to lift? A look at the rich, older women in California may answer that one. Half-starved, anorexic figures, they have faces that look like they have been pulled to within an inch of their lives. There is no expression and no trace of the life that has been lived – just vapid, smooth, perfection.

Chapter Seven

Society

Imagine a candlelit dinner for two in a romantic restaurant. A sixty-five-year-old man is entertaining a fabulous-looking twenty-five-year-old woman. Now look at the table over the other side of the restaurant where a sixty-five-year-old woman is having dinner with a fabulous twenty-five-year-old man. Would you assume the young man was the woman's lover? Or would you think he was her son? And if he is her lover, do you feel the same about them as the first couple?

In this chapter, I looked at the way society treats older women. Did women feel that society has changed since feminism? Did they feel an identifiable group, or were they very much individuals? Did they want society to change or were they quite happy with the way older women are treated? What about institutions like the media, politics and the Church? Did they feel like full participants in the body politic, or were they stuck on the sidelines?

Society has changed almost beyond recognition in the lifetime of the women in this book. Women in their seventies and eighties had their lives pretty well mapped out for them, they knew how they were supposed to dress, where they were in the rigid social hierarchy, lives that were not that different from the ones their mothers lived.

The values of society were unquestioned, that was how life was and women had their clear place in the model. In return for keeping their place, they were looked after and protected; men would open doors for them (but only ones that didn't matter), walk on the outside of them in the street and generally play the role of chevalier servant. Weakness in women was associated with femininity – women who wanted to live their own lives were regarded as freaks (look at the way gay women felt obliged to dress in full male regalia in the past) and had the greatest threat of all held over them, that they would not find husbands.

Women now in their fifties and sixties were the first to have access to financial independence and dependable contraception. The rule book had to be rewritten.

The last thirty years has seen a massive readjustment between the sexes which has been painful for both sides. While men have often felt threatened and lost when they are no longer welcome guides and protectors, women too have felt confused by the new possibilities and constraints. If a woman doesn't change her name when she gets married, what do they call the children? Does she want doors opened for her sometimes, always, never? When are compliments from men agreeable, and when do they constitute sexual harassment?

Changes in people's private lives have been mirrored by social upheaval. The seventies saw a rash of profiles in the press about 'firsts' – the first woman to drive a long-distance lorry, run a restaurant business, present the news. Those stories seem old fashioned now, but notable firsts are still slow in coming. The first woman speaker of the House of Commons, the first head of the Secret Services, the first ordained woman priest are recent changes.

Conservative men have retaliated by hunkering down. Last year I went to do an interview in an exclusive man's club, only to be asked politely to use the stairs reserved for ladies, not the magnificent main sweep (what did they think I would do, pee on the carpet?).

There are mutterings from more liberal men about having cake and eating it, which is understandable when they have had the cake to themselves all these years. Of course, it is important for women not to fall into the trap of becoming pale imitations of men. But that is where the difficulty lies; we are in the process of working out new codes of practice at work and new ways of balancing power in relationships. With more than two thousand years of history of doing it one way, it's hardly surprising that readjustment will cause resentment and retrenching by the diehard defenders of the old order.

But the new order also offers advantages to men. They no longer have to be the strong, silent types who feel unnable to show their feelings. Men have as much to gain as women from the new partnership.

Katherine

Fifty-three. After many years bringing up a family, she has come into her own in the work place. She is a classic woman returner, holding down a highly responsible job in a television company. She is angry about the raw deal older women get. Perhaps because she doesn't look her age, she is aware of the value judgements placed by others on older women.

I get so pissed off about the way society looks at older women, because they will talk about women of a certain age; what the hell does that mean? They group all people from the age of forty onwards as oldies and despise them for some reason, it's very shortsighted. There are growing numbers of us, we're getting more and more affluent, things are going to have to change.

Maybe it's something to do with the menopause –

nature says you're not any good any more, and society is just reflecting that, all you're good for is just bringing up your grandchildren, being the matriarch, the pivot of the family, making the Sunday roast. It must be quite disturbing for society, looking at this monstrous brigade of women standing up for their rights a bit more.

I don't act like a grandmother, maybe I'm fighting society's image of me in that way. We're not all little grey-haired people sitting down with our knitting! Women like myself will change things, but at the moment it's still very patronising out there.

Katherine belongs to the generation of women that has achieved economic independence through working for most of their lives, with time off to bring up children. These women are now reaching the pinnacle of their careers, the time when men at the same stage would be invited to take up directorships and other key positions of influence. But while spotting a woman at the Institute of Directors (apart from the staff) still feels like the sighting of a rare lesser spotted grebe, while the House of Lords still considers women unfit to take up hereditary peerages, and the great and the good are still largely chosen from the ranks of men, society is losing a swathe of key highfliers.

Brenda

Fifty-four. She is a woman returner too. After happily staying at home to bring up her children and loving being a mum, her husband's redundancy meant she had to find work. Now she works for a medium-sized computer firm and is somewhat bemused at her new role. She is modest about her achievements.

Society treats women better now. My one beef is clothes. I go shopping with my daughters, and I like all of their clothes, but I can't wear them. They're too sexy and too young and I suppose I'm the greatest one for saying,

'Look at her, anyone would think . . .!' so I have this thing about what people would say about me, about not looking like mutton dressed as lamb.

There is nothing in the shops, there's no trendy stuff for women of our age, they don't seem to cater for us. My husband, he's a great one for, 'If you want to wear it, have it', and then I'll probably realise three weeks later that he didn't like it! He'd tell me if he doesn't like something, like he hates track suits, they're so baggy.

It's frustrating, I feel I can't buy any trendy clothes, I'm stopped by the idea of what people might think. I'm getting a bit better, I really am, what I'll do is buy something and try it out on holiday and then if I have the courage to wear it on holiday, I'll wear it at home. We've been friends with similar sorts of people for a very long time, and we've stayed in the same house. We're known with a certain image and you're stuck with it. I am getting better, but when I started work full time I had to be two different people sometimes, the person I wanted to be at work, wasn't the Brenda they knew, so that was difficult.

Brenda has a split identity. When I met her she was dressed in the working woman's uniform, smart suit and feminine blouse. Her image at home is stylish and comfortable, but it's when the two worlds collide that she has difficulty reconciling her public and private personas. The idea that this creative, self-confident woman might worry about what the neighbours thought of her outfits shows how much peer pressure women still feel. The ideal at home is not to stand out, make a fuss, seem different from anyone else. Of course, this clashes head on with what is required from the working woman, who needs to get herself noticed to get on. Brenda has come up with a clever way to get round her shyness at wearing trendy clothes at home, she tries them out incognito in the house or on holiday. She feels she needs to reconcile her own desire with what she imagines are the commandments laid down by her immediate peer group. The sinners are cast into the outer darkness amid much gnashing of teeth.

Joan

Fifty-two. She is an evangelical Christian who has remained celibate for religious reasons. She is involved in her community, with a responsible job in local government planning. She has a deep commitment to her beliefs, but is not unquestioning.

Older women don't have a voice, although things are changing. The power structures are such that it's still very difficult for women to hold their own, and make their voices and their values heard. That is certainly my experience at work. One still feels like a token woman on certain committees and in certain circles. If you take a weekend conference, like the one I've just been on, there were ninety of us from all over Europe, and it was very noticeable that the real power is still held by the men, even though the women do most of the work. In the media there's not enough representation of women on good panels like *Question Time*, they're very heavily dominated by men. I don't think older women get any good press at all, I can't think of any good older role models.

Women are also an invisible force within the Church. The Church and women is a very fraught subject! I'm an Anglican, evangelical Anglican. I feel very ambivalent about women's ordination, in fact I find myself disagreeing with the hard evangelical line. I am for women's ordination and would want to differ from some of my friends in that.

The evangelical community as a whole, says a lot about women's ministry, but hands over no real power to them and allows them very little influence. Women are allowed a ministry but it has to be within the framework that men have set up, so they are an invisible workforce that works extremely hard.

*Joan shows the changes that have taken place in conservative religious
circles in the last fifteen years. Although an evangelical Christian,
who has remained celibate because she disapproves of sex before
marriage, her views on women's role in the Church are radical.
Women have always been the glue that held the Church together; they
attend services, but also clean the churches, arrange the flowers and
generally make sure the parish ticks over. In the Church of England
women have pushed for and obtained ordination, though not without
an unprecedented rear-guard action which showed the extent of
misogyny masquerading as theology within the Church. In the
Roman Catholic Church, many women are demanding that their
role be recognised. Girl altar servers were the first step, and although
it was predicted that civilised society as we know it would come to an
end, life has continued much as before. But women still have a long
way to go, as can be seen by the huge protest against the use of inclusive
language (not automatically using 'he' or 'man' in prayers).*

Rose

*Eighty-four. She has lived in the same area all her life and has a
strong sense of community. She always went out to work, doing
several cleaning jobs, while bringing up her family and looking
after an invalid husband. We discuss the forthcoming elections and
she is up on all the main political stories. A Labour voter all her
life, she has a strong sense of social justice. She manages, just, on
the basic state pension.*

Standards have really changed now. We're much too
bothered about sex – look at all these top people selling
these books, millionaires! I think that should be stopped
because it's encouraging people. I mean look at the MPs
and the Royal Family. They're in charge of us, we've got
to look up to them, you get someone licking someone else's
toes, that is disgusting! All these MPs as well, they
shouldn't be in charge of the country, telling us what
to do and what not to do.

Women are taking over and being the bosses. That's good because I do think the women have been bossed about enough, from way back. It's good that men are helping more about the house, because years ago the father was the bully, the Victorian style of doing things. But now a man will listen to a woman, and together they'll look after the children. They grow up nice then.

My great granddaughter, she's twelve, she knows everything about it, a very sensible girl, she knows more than I know now! In a way I'm pleased, these day she can protect herself a bit, she knows more. I hope she'll have a happy marriage. It's a different world completely.

Rose has seen enormous social changes in her lifetime. The class system, although still strong, has nowhere near the power it did when she was a girl. The media has given up the craven attitude it used to have towards the powers that be, indeed it sometimes seems bent on proving that all institutions are riddled with embezzlers and adulterers.

Ordinary people no longer accept the idea of the rich man in his castle, the beggar at the gate. Questioning the role of the monarchy – brought about in large part by people realising that the young royals misbehaved like anyone else – was unthinkable until recently. The establishment is still fighting back, but ideas like the dis-establishment of the Church, the Royal Family paying income tax, and the equal opportunities bill, which would have seemed revolu-tionary even twenty years ago, are today seen by people like Rose as the first steps in the break-up of the class system towards a fairer society.

Annie

Fifty-six. As a gay woman before the feminist revolution, her perspective on sexuality and society has always included an acute sense of being different and secret. This put tremendous strain on her at times and she has suffered from depression.

We were mostly closeted of course, except to one or two lesbian couples. I wasn't out to my family, I wasn't out to anybody in the office. When you get left, it's particularly awful, because you go to work, you go to the shops and you can't cry and say my partner's just gone off and left me. Even though I think my sister must have known what sort of relationship it was, we'd certainly never spoken about it. I certainly would never to my mother, my mother would have killed me.

If you're someone who hasn't been married and isn't in a relationship, another people can look upon you as a totally asexual being. I have actually had more sexual experience than my sister has, and more than quite a lot of people I know. But while you're not saying, 'I'm a lesbian', they can and do assume that you're an old maid. But as soon as you come out, they look upon you as nothing else but a sexual being.

The area of sexual politics has been transformed beyond recognition in Annie's lifetime. Today a young, gay woman would not grow up in her twenties believing she was the only gay woman in London. Gay women have won the right to adopt children, have artificial insemination and have their own clubs and publishing houses. Work is a different matter. Though lesbianism has always been more easily accepted than male homosexuality, many gay women still find it difficult to come out to their colleagues at work, fearing prejudice and hostility. And the fact that many straight women in public office, like the police force, who complain about unfair treatment are immediately branded lesbians, as though that weakened their argument, shows how far we still have to go.

Elizabeth

Seventy-seven. She has brought up a big family with a difficult husband who seems incapable of showing her any affection. She has not a trace of bitterness about her.

Society doesn't treat us terribly well, I think we are still a nuisance, we take up their time, we're slower at doing things.

In a society that prizes speed, from faxes to quiz shows, anyone who is beginning to slow down is treated with contempt. Society puts a premium on anything that can save us time, from convenience foods to home gadgets, but what are we to do with all those spare hours we've saved by microwaving a pre-cooked meal?

Judith

Sixty-two. She recently retired, though she has been asked to go back part time, which she admits she rather likes, as it shows they can't manage completely without her. She is very aware of the importance of economic independence to women of her generation.

Things have changed quite a bit for my generation and are still changing. Single older women, especially, who like me have worked all their lives, are much better off financially, even for married women it must be different now. We are more secure financially than our mothers were.

Otherwise I'm not sure. A woman who is widowed and left on her own is often more isolated than she used to be, communities are not so close-knit, there is not necessarily the network of families and friends of a similar age.

I'd like to see attitudes towards older women changing, but I think they are slowly. Society often sees women's sexuality as linked to fertility, so if you're not fertile, you're not sexual and one is no longer any use, but I don't agree with that. Maybe that's the male view, and that should change. Men are afraid of women now because they have much more control over these things.

Now the first generations of independent women are retiring, in good health, with pensions, they are searching for a new role.

Women in their sixties can look forward to many more years of active life than men, and they will not want to retire from positions of influence to do what their mothers and grandmothers did.

Clare

Fifty-six. She is married to a pillar of the community who has had serious problems with alcohol, but she has stuck by him.

I hope these days society doesn't think of women as 'post-menopausal'. I have a friend, with a pig of a husband, who said, 'Well that's it, all you're useful for is carrying the shopping basket'. But I don't think, on the whole, men think of us like that. Post-menopausal women do tend to be lumped together by the media – if you're sixty you're virtually geriatric and you are lumped at fifty with women of eighty. You're thought of as not having very much of a life after sixty. It is gradually changing as people discuss things more. I mean I wouldn't have dreamed of discussing this sort of thing with my mother, but I can with you.

Until I began this book, I had never thought of older women as individuals, anyone beyond sixty-five fell into the file marked 'old'. The media is puzzled by women who don't conform to what society imagines a woman of sixty or seventy should look like, or if they behave in a way it considers eccentric. But many women reported that menopause had allowed them to behave and dress the way they wanted, without the pressures of society for the first time in their lives.

Alice

Sixty. She is very image conscious, as she is the boss in a medium-sized company. After two unhappy marriages she is now back with her first husband. Financial security is a priority because her husband has amassed debts which she is paying off. She is worried about the future.

I'm more self-assured as I've got older, that's age rather than menopause. Society views older women positively as long as they are dressed well. Look at the magazines, they don't look at anyone who is dowdy and grey-haired. I'm very conscious of that. I'm not going to be a quiet little old lady, certainly not, I'm going to be kicking and screaming and fighting.

How far should women conform to the role society expects of them? They will certainly have an easier passage if they do conform, but how will things ever change if we accept the status quo? Even the words society applies to older women are full of significance. Think woman and grey. Now think man and grey. Suddenly words like distinguished, silver, sexy come to mind.

Madeleine

Seventy-three. She has had a long and happy marriage and has worked as a counsellor. She admits to having been very pretty and getting a lot of attention when younger. She radiates contentment and joy.

When you're older, for some people it's as though you're not there. It's happened to me, when you're standing at the counter and nobody seems to notice that you are there. I will not be cowed, I will speak up and not be pushed around by younger people. You're written off. I can remember when I was twenty saying, 'I'm sure that people, when they are sixty, will be happy to just go, they've done it all, what else can they contribute!'

As you get older you move that deadline, literally. I don't think you'll ever alter young people because they live in a world of their own and I don't wish to encroach on that world, I wouldn't fit in and they feel awkward in mine.

The invisibility factor can be useful for older women, it allows them to get on with their lives in peace. The danger is that younger people get impatient with the slower rhythms of older women, thinking their time is not as precious. Madeleine recognises the two worlds of youth and maturity, we just need to learn to speak each other's language.

Mavis

Seventy-three. She is still sexually active, and has recently had a happy affair with a forty-four-year-old man. She has a very positive view about herself, still working part time and doing volunteer work.

We're not all crabby old dears. There are a lot of older women who would be very happy to have a sexual relationship if they found one. Why should sex stop at fifty? Why should it? I'm sure that women can go on a lot longer than men, but then a lot of older women find younger men.

The difference today is that people talk about sex all the time, there's no need for it. You can talk about it openly, and that's a very good thing but it depends how you talk about it. Some of the young people, their language is awful, the way they describe what they are doing, I don't think it's necessary. Nothing has changed a great deal.

Society ignores us as older women, we don't exist, I'm a non-person. No one cares about you, no one worries about you, you have to look after yourself and stand on your own two feet.

In a society where youth is God, older women must fit in where they can. I found myself surprised that a woman of seventy-three would still be able to have an affair with a man in his forties, although the reverse would have seemed more acceptable in society's eyes.

Jenny

Fifty-four. She has two sons with learning difficulties and a fourteen-year-old daughter. She has started dating again after her divorce and is determined not to be stereotyped as an older woman. She is a teacher in a large comprehensive.

Society thinks I should settle down and be quiet, I've got a child to bring up and a job and that should be enough. I know people think 'She's lucky really, she comes home and does her knitting in the evening!' It's because on the whole, the world seems to be made up of couples and their cosy little lives, and singles do feel outside of that. But does it matter what they think, do we need to let them know that we are not leading lives like that?

I've got a lot of single women friends, divorced or widowed. We lead a gay social life. As there will be more and more single women, they're not just going to stick at home. We're a force to be reckoned with, there are more and more of us. It's almost like a secret society of older women! People at work, I can't think any of them imagine that I lead the life that I do, not at all! I'm sure they just think that I come home, cook tea, watch telly and go to work again the next day. I'm sure they have no idea of my real life.

Jenny represents the rising generation of menopausal women who refuse to be pigeon-holed like their older sisters. I'd love to meet her when she turns eighty, still not watching telly or knitting!

Sally

Fifty-two. She is conscious of being more sexual since menopause and society's disapproval.

Every word about menopause seems to be scathing, 'Oh, she's on the change', or 'She's menopausal' said in that particular tone of voice. Every word that relates to the womb is pejorative; if you look at a woman in a city, imagine a woman on the tube having a hot flush, people reading their newspapers on the way to the office, she'd be treated like she was barmy! So therefore women suppress it.

There are fields full of women put out to grass. I know women in their nineties who are strong, forceful and ignored by the world. Menopause should be ignored or absorbed, I don't think there should be such a hullaballoo about it, but within that, it should be noticed that women have alarming symptoms. Not bleeding is great, it's a delight after all these years.

If you think of a lined man, you would say he was distinguished, a distinguished woman is not synonymous with a sexual woman. I find that upsetting. I know a few men who say they don't mind wrinkled women, but it's unusual.

If you watch Dame Edna and her sidekick Madge on television and see people roaring with laughter, that's how people see older women, figures of fun or pathos, or just plain dotty. Women are a hidden army. The idea of an older woman having desire is alien to a lot of people. That image of a woman is insidious and disgusting, I don't really understand why people find it funny.

The fields of women put out to grass are beginning to question the role that society has prepared for them. Dame Edna, a man in drag, humiliates the menopausal woman — would we laugh if it were a real woman? Or at a woman in drag making fun of a man in his sixties?

Maud

Seventy-eight. She is very conscious of her appearance. She is a smart, sparky woman who likes the company of younger women because she often finds women her own age unwilling to talk about issues seriously.

The average picture of an older woman is someone who is slightly bent with white hair. Sometimes I look at them, and think no way would any man consider having an affair with her. I often look at them with a certain amount of pity. A woman always needs to have some sort of confidence in her sexuality and it looks to me like a lot of them have nothing. A lot of them are quite happy to have lost it maybe. Also they get into gangs with one another and there's a lot of comfort in that, I don't think I want to do that really.

I wonder if some older women feel they have missed out because of television, this impression that everybody is having this free sexual thing.

Maud admits that she generally prefers the company of men to women because she finds men are more intellectual. For women of her generation to come out with their opinions, or hold the floor in debate, was considered unseemly and unfeminine. Maud still suffers from the prejudice that women getting into gangs are gossiping or doing something not worthwhile. That seems to suggest that the presence of a man is needed to stamp the occasion with the imprimatur of intellectual rigour. But anyone who has ever overheard a group of men chatting in the pub about the best way to get from point A to point B will know that they are not all up to discussing the first law of thermodynamics.

Dot

Seventy. Dot feels she has finally sorted herself out since meno-pause, despite managing a large hospital department for many years.

It's very difficult to think of yourself as an older woman, so the way society looks at us doesn't bother me one scrap. It's like water off a duck's back. I don't know when I shall ever come to terms with it! I probably would if I were incapacitated, but I am far too active to see it. I don't conform at all, I don't want to and see no reason to. I act like myself, not my age, I can't see why we should turn a corner and become something. For one thing, I believe we are given opportunities to start a different life after retirement, and it never stops and why should it?

Chapter Eight

The new generation

Most of this book has involved women looking back on their lives; recounting their marriages and relationships, looking at how menopause changed priorities, comparing how they felt about themselves then and now. I wanted to build a picture of menopause, and how it affects women of different ages. But I also wanted them to look forwards, to the rising generations.

What did women in their seventies and eighties feel about the future as represented by the lives of younger women? Some of their own daughters would soon be approaching menopause, had they given them advice on how to weather any storms that might be lying in wait for them? Many older women in this book were brought up by parents who could never have imagined the changes that have taken place in society, the opportunities available to women, the changes in relationships, men taking more responsibility for child care. So how did they see the future?

Had they brought up their children and grandchildren differently? What did they think of the rising generations? Were they envious of the freedoms of younger women? Did they think that those freedoms had gone too far? Would they prefer to belong to the younger generations? What did they think of the younger generations' views of them? Did they approve of more awareness and freedom in sexual matters? What had they allowed their children to do? What hopes did they have for their granddaughters?

Older women with children are in no doubt that life is better for women now than when they were growing up. Not just in the realm of job opportunities, but also in home life as well. Women can now expect to be happy in their relationships, a notion quite alien to older generations. You got married and if it didn't work out, that was tough. They admired the fact that younger women have access to divorce to escape brutish behaviour from husbands.

Younger women are better informed about sex, too. They no longer get married knowing absolutely nothing about life behind the bedroom door, and I couldn't find a single woman in her seventies and eighties who longed for the so-called good old days of ignorance. Many of them spoke of wasted opportunities with husbands they had loved, but who had no more idea of sexual technique than they did. Many were wistful when looking at their daughters and granddaughters and thinking about the pleasure that might have been.

But relationships are not just about sex; older women are envious of the closeness visible in younger couples. This closeness comes from the liberation from gender roles where people are not so entrenched in 'appropriate' behaviour for men and women. When older women described their husbands of several decades, I was often left with the impression that they had been virtual strangers, despite living under the same roof for years.

Of course the biggest change of all is that women now can choose not to have children. This has left them free to direct their own lives, free from the economic dependence on men. Mothers and grandmothers admire the new young women; their zest for life, their freedom, their sense that they can do anything they want with their lives.

They had all been conscious, in bringing up their own children, that they wanted more affection in their lives, not the cold distance that many of them had suffered. They wanted their daughters to know about sex; even the youngest woman, only forty-seven, felt it imperative for her to break the link of repression that had been forged down the generations. Although she found it difficult to talk to her daughter about sex, she is proud that the resulting openness between them has allowed the daughter to have more rounded, natural relationships.

They look ahead to the marriages and relationships that would be made in the next century, and are optimistic for the granddaughters who now come to them for advice.

Alice

Sixty. She has two sons and married twice, now living again with her first husband. She is very sceptical about men and relationships.

I don't envy the younger generation their sexual freedom, I envy them their youth, they've got a life ahead of them.

Alice looks back on her life and regrets the path she chose. By returning to her first husband, who has saddled her with debts, and whom she describes as a waster, it's as though she is walking backwards through her life, trying to recapture the excitement. But what guarantees are there that she would not make the same mistakes?

Elizabeth

Seventy-seven. She is closer to her children and grandchildren than her husband. She is an affectionate woman who has always been surrounded by the younger generation. She had two children in her forties and was menopausal while they were still pre-school.

I'm a matriarchal figure, very much so, having run a large family and having had to be the fount of all wisdom for them. Even now the older grandchildren feel they can come and talk to me about things they can't talk to their parents about. I do like that. Perhaps that has given me more wisdom, certainly a lot more tolerance. I still get on extremely well with the very young grandchildren and great grandchildren, they don't seem to be put off by me at all!

My children's marriages were very different from mine, that is just a generational thing. The girls particularly are much more expressive, they wouldn't accept the things I accepted. They expect their husbands to be loving and kind and have a physical relationship with them.

On the whole there is a loving relationship between them all, after all my eldest son is now a grandfather and that marriage has lasted well. They've all stayed with their partners, I hope I did something right in bringing them up.

My daughters knew more than I ever did at quite a young age! My eldest daughter, she talks to me much more, she's coming up for fifty. She was most worried because her husband had heart trouble, he was on all kinds of pills and she was most upset because he had lost his sex drive. She did tell me that they had always had an extremely satisfactory physical relationship and it really was a trial for her. Don't laugh will you, they got exotic films! [*She roars with laughter.*] I approved of anything that would keep her marriage stable and happy. That was the most important thing.

My eldest daughter, who is a very warm and loving person, she's the most physical of them all, she may have strayed once or twice, but it has never been anything very serious.

I don't think I envy their freedom, particularly my grandchildren's generation, they have made an awful lot of problems for themselves. We had set rules, we knew how we should behave and how far we could go, which I don't think we found terribly inhibiting because I don't think, on the whole, we had any desire to break loose in that way. This present generation, what rules have they got?

It's very good that women do have better sexual relationships now. There's nothing wrong in expecting to have good sex, as long as they don't cause trouble. I object to this business of them just sleeping around with any Tom, Dick and Harry or breaking up families over it. But there's no reason why women shouldn't expect more, her desires are just as great as a man's and she's entitled to have them satisfied. I should think if you do have a good physical relationship it must be rather wonderful.

Elizabeth shows no bitterness at the appalling treatment she has had to put up with from her husband; she is simply glad that her daughters and granddaughters will not have to suffer as she has done. Elizabeth's treatment is the best argument for social change, though she is not convinced that the freedoms of my generation are wholly positive.

Katherine

Fifty-three. She wonders if the sexual difficulties in her own marriage have affected her children.

My eldest daughter is married, my youngest daughter lives with a guy. The youngest is extremely happy sexually, more sexually than in other ways, listening to her talk. My elder daughter isn't as happy sexually, she doesn't actually tell me, she's more embarrassed to talk about that sort of thing to me than my younger daughter, always has been. I can see the same pattern in her life as in mine, and that's very strange. She loves her husband absolutely, he's a lovely chap, but she's not that happy sexually. She's always been very keen on sex, right from the beginning, as soon as she was sixteen she said, 'What do I do now I'm legal?' She's had a lot of lovers, so she's probably expecting more and they've only been married five years or so.

Katherine is surprised that her daughter seems to have reproduced her parents' relationship with her husband in her own marriage. But patterns of behaviour can be reproduced down the generations. Elizabeth clearly brought her daughters up to expect more than she received, but Katherine seems to have given her daughter different messages. The idea of there being a legal dividing line for sex, beyond which promiscuous behaviour is acceptable seems strange. As we know from Dot's experience, having lots of lovers doesn't necessarily mean having good sex, or having a high opinion of oneself.

Rose

Eighty-four. She is from a generation which grew up in complete ignorance of sex. She is very keen on the idea of the family network and has photos of her family throughout her flat.

The young people of today can enjoy their sex, that's great, definitely, because nature's made it. God gave us the gift to have sex, not just to have children, but a feeling that naturally came to you, because everybody doesn't have children.

I should imagine that my children's marriages are better, but you never know, some of them might go and see someone else, or you know, fancy someone else. I don't know, they never talk to me about it. I was brought up in that way, we never conversed about sex or anything like that. I didn't tell my sons about it, and even now, if something comes on the telly and it's to do with sex, and nowadays you see them performing sex, my son he doesn't know what to do, I don't know what to do and I get very, very embarrassed. I make out to get up, or he does. I'm not embarrassed at all talking to you, because you put me at ease and also being a woman . . . I couldn't talk to a man.

I don't think my husband talked to them at all either. It's only come on in the last twenty years. I've got two grandchildren of thirty-six and two of thirty-three and they're married with children. Their marriages are very different, you can tell when they laugh and joke in company about different sex things, which we wouldn't have dared said. It's best to know, that's what they should have done with us, years and years ago.

Rose is an important witness to the change in women's lives in the twentieth century. Meeting her feels like shaking hands with the past. It's vital to look back with clear eyes, to have the testimony of women like Rose, if we are to appreciate how much better our lives are, and how much better still our daughter's lives can be.

Judith

Sixty-two. She has worked with young people for many years and is not sure that all the changes are good. She has no children herself.

I do envy the younger generation, up to a point, but I also feel quite sad for them in many ways. Although sex is so much easier for them, how dangerous it is also for them, because of AIDS in particular, and also other sexually transmitted diseases. But yes, in some ways I do envy them, in that when I think back to one or two of my friends when I was younger, maybe it would have been nice to have tried the sexual experience to see whether or not it would have worked or we would have been compatible.

Clare

Fifty-six. She has a no-nonsense approach to sex despite difficulties in her own marriage. She believes that marriage must be worked at and certain things just put up with. She is worried that history may be repeating itself.

I think my children do have good physical relationships. Unfortunately my elder daughter has been separated for two years. Obviously I told them about sex. The elder one got married very young, I think it was an escape from mother and father being divorced and feeling a bit torn apart and her marriage was very happy for eleven years. It almost looks as though she is following mother's pattern in a way but I don't like to think that. She was very happy, she's got two lovely children, she's a very well balanced girl. She was eighteen when she got married, her husband was twelve years older, rather domineering in a way and she accepted exactly what he said, and did what he did. Then she developed and she's her own person now and they parted. She was attracted to somebody else, but it didn't work out, that set things off. The other one is happily married, I think they do have a good sex life, somehow you can tell.

Clare is worried that her daughter, too, may be following an unsuccessful path in relationships, the difference is that they can talk about it, whereas Clare would never have been able to discuss her sexual problems with her own mother.

Caroline

Seventy-three. She is convinced that her own marital problems – she split up with her first husband when he went off with someone else, married a concentration camp survivor with four teenage children and when he died, she eventually remarried her first husband – have had a knock-on effect on her children.

I was able to talk to my children about sex because our marriage was very good then, when they were eight, nine, ten, eleven, twelve. They were always asking questions and we were very free, everybody went to the bathroom together, bathed together, nobody bothered, it was always very, very, easy. It was very different from my upbringing.

It's no accident that the boy has a very happy marriage and the other three have very difficult marriages. The girls were parted from their father and that mattered. My son is very happy in his marriage, I like her very much.

My eldest daughter was the last to get married. She had a big affair with a married man and he left his home and they lived together. He was my age, it was very difficult, I couldn't really see it working out, but they seemed terribly happy together, but he was dallying over the question of divorce. She had an invitation to go to America, so she decided she would go and let him get on with it. Well what did he do, he went straight back to his wife! It was the most ghastly shock to her, she was terribly unhappy over that. She was in her mid-twenties.

A few years later, she wanted to get married and she did find someone. It's a marriage that really has to be worked at; he's not an easy person, he's a very stubborn man, he's been very unloved in his own family, so he's needed tremendous boosting. He's very exhausting to live with. He comes in and bangs all the cupboard doors, it is a very tempestuous marriage.

Her twin married a teacher, they've got one girl. I think Jonathan has got a very low sex drive, he doesn't want it very much, he's always been like that – it's more or less a miracle that the little girl was born. She's never had any other children because she says your husband's got to make love to you if you're going to have children. It's been

a very, very difficult time for her because she has a much
stronger sex drive and I think it has been a real struggle.
They're very attached to one another, I know he loves her
dearly but he can't express it in a way that she wants him
to express it. She hasn't had affairs with other people,
they've had a lot of help, and she's just learned to live with
it. People learn to put up with those situations.

My fourth daughter is another traumatic story. She had
a baby with a boy who pushed off just before it was born.
Then she married this chap who had just come out of
prison for manslaughter. He came back and found his
second wife of six weeks in bed with another man and took
a carving knife to this fellow. It's a pretty extreme way of
dealing with things, and I certainly didn't want my
daughter to marry him. They lived together for a time.
What she sees in him I simply don't know, they have two
children of twelve and nine. They are still married, just –
they have had fearful ups and downs, she's been to see a
solicitor three times but she always takes him back. He has
been violent with her, and I feel with anybody who knocks
his wife about, you never know how bad it is going to be.

They were threatened with the bailiffs a few months
ago. She then went for an injunction to keep him away
and she got it for three months and we thought, 'Thank,
goodness, this really is it this time', but not a bit of it, she's
had him back again. There's some co-dependence there,
they can't manage without each other and they can't live
together, so I don't know how it will all end. I worry
about the grandchildren, he's no role model as a father.

Often you skip a generation, your children don't come
to you so much, but your grandchildren do. I'm beginning to feel that, even my twelve-year-old granddaughter
said to me, 'Could I ask your advice Granny?' There's this
boy at school and he'd written her a note, he said he
fancied her and could she fancy him? And she didn't
really, she liked him as a friend. Rather sweet! I said, 'If I

were you, I'd write a little note back and thank him very much for his note, and say that you like him as a friend but don't feel you want it to go any further than that'. I was rather touched that she came to me. I think twelve is a bit young, it's rather a pity, their childhood is shortened.

On the whole it's rather more difficult for this generation. It's right that things should come out into the open and we can talk about all these things more freely. On the other hand, it can also be a bit damaging too, there was a code of behaviour and discipline round our lives. Ours wasn't anything like as strict as our parents. I feel that we hit it about right, our generation, you could talk about sex and be free with your boyfriends, but there was a certain code of behaviour which was a good thing which added to the stability of life, there is no stability now.

Caroline raises an important question: how far are we responsible for the lives our children lead? She has felt tremendous guilt that her marital problems have provided a bad model for her daughters. Yet her generation also had difficult marriages, they just put up with them. Problems are out in open these days. One daughter has married a difficult man, but the accounts of older women in this book are littered with difficult men, another has sexual problems, but that is not so strange. The daughter who has married the man just out of prison is more worrying. Caroline feels she may be repeating her own coping patterns. But ultimately, we are all responsible for our own lives and we can't blame our parents for all our mistakes.

Madeleine

Seventy-three. She has the happiest marriage of the whole group, her face lights up when she talks of her husband of forty-six years. She is open and affectionate.

Your generation thinks they've discovered sex, every new generation does. Even I find it a bit odd, thinking of someone in their eighties, so I can understand someone in their forties thinking, 'Oh she doesn't need it at her age!'

My son didn't wish to know about sex. I remember he was going abroad on a school trip, he was about thirteen and I tried to talk about it and he said I didn't have to say a word! My daughter was very open and always wanted to know everything and her friends had mothers who didn't like to talk about it so they used to come back with her and put the questions. I was a science teacher then so we used to sit and have discussions about sex and feelings. I used to say to them, 'You say that won't happen to you, you won't let a boy do that, but your body takes over, you have to be prepared for your body to over-rule everything you have been thinking. You have to be much stronger to be able to say "no" and come away from it.' They always used to come and whisper, 'You ask your mum!'

My son has always been a bit uptight, he doesn't show his emotions. He says, 'You know I love you', and I say, 'No I don't, how do I know?' Whereas my daughter is very open and affectionate and fortunately has married a man who is the same. Unfortunately, my son married a woman who is the same as he is, rather cold, looks after the children well, but there's just that bit of distance. Before that he had a lovely, warm, smiley woman. He needed warming up I thought. But he's happy.

Good, accurate information about sex is vital for adolescents. And while sex education in schools has advanced beyond recognition in the last twenty years, it's still difficult for teenagers to ask embarrassing questions in confidence, in front of a classroom of their peers. Madeleine provided an essential safe haven, a place where a small group of young women could ask questions and know they would get good information and that they would be treated seriously.

Mavis

Seventy-three. She was pregnant with her daughter as her mother had a late baby during menopause. She has a strong sense of family connection. She is slightly impatient with the younger generation for the loss of standards in appearance and behaviour.

My daughter was married for twenty-four years and she had a very good relationship. He came home one day and said he had met someone else. I had known for a long time that there was something not quite right between them, but she was heartbroken at the time.

She recently married again and I remember saying to her, 'I know that you didn't have a good sex life with your husband, but you are going to have to learn to enjoy it now'. I had a gut feeling about it. I'm very close to my daughter and we've always been able to discuss things. Her new husband is fifty and she says that she is having a wonderful sex life.

My granddaughter is living with a man, I think she's got a good sexual relationship. A lot of young people today, they don't take enough time to get to know each other. With a one-night stand, if you see someone you fancy and wonder what he would be like in bed, if you get him into bed, he is probably useless, or two minutes and back to square one again!

Although her daughter's first marriage didn't work out, Mavis is a great optimist. She sensed that things would be different with the second husband and was close enough to her daughter to be able to speak frankly to her. Her experience in sex makes her disapprove of one-night stands, not on moral grounds but because they are likely to be disappointing.

Jenny

Fifty-four. She has two older sons with learning difficulties and a younger daughter. She is a single parent who likes to have fun with her children but is conscious of the need for her own space. She is determined that her own disastrous relationship with her mother should not go on down through the generations. She is dating again after the break-up of her marriage.

My children laugh at me, 'Who is tonight then mother!' I'm always very honest about where I am going and what I am doing. It's part of their lives as well, I'm bringing them home. My youngest is fourteen, just at the age when she is beginning to be interested. She's a bit mixed up, I haven't had a serious relationship for two years, she didn't like that at all, she was a little monkey when I was going out with Charlie and did everything she could do to put a spoke in the wheels.

Dad had gone and here was her mum going out, she wanted me to herself very much. I don't know how she would react if I had a really close, serious relationship again, although we do talk about it. When she has a boyfriend herself, she'll find it easier to accept. But the roles are reversed almost. I bring the men home to see if the children will like them and approve!

I didn't think I would still be doing that at my age. It makes a difference if the children don't like them. My youngest has suffered quite a lot with the break-up, and I wouldn't want to add to that at all. But at the end of the day, she is going to be eighteen in four years time and leaving home and she won't want me. To a certain extent you can't consider your children all the time. If I met someone who was right and she didn't like him, tough, because in the end, I've got a long time on my own and she's leaving. I do try to consider her a bit, but I've got to think of the future.

New patterns of relationships for mothers mean that they may well be dating and having relationships again at the same time as their daughters. This brings problems of etiquette, a mother can't confide in a daughter in the same way she would a friend. What if the daughter disapproves of her mother's choice? Freedom will always bring complications. In the past, women often simply gave up on the idea of relationships and lived through their children. Modern women like Jenny feel they too, have a right to happiness.

Florrie

Eighty-four. She was brought up in fear of what the neighbours would say. Her own two marriages have been happy and she now has a live-in boyfriend much younger than herself. Her two children were born when she was in her forties.

My parents always wanted us to conform, so I wanted to let my children have what I didn't have; freedom. I think both my children have happy marriages. My son married someone with three children; she'd been abandoned, left high and dry. We weren't awfully keen on her at first, but she's turned out well, done him a lot of good, they have a daughter.

I didn't encourage my children to sleep with people, but I didn't stand in their way, I guessed what was going on. That's the big change for their generation, they admit it's going on. It's no good being hateful to your children, they're only doing something natural.

Florrie is proud that her children have been able to enjoy freedoms that she never had. The fear of neighbours, who secured the tight network of social control, no longer holds sway. Florrie was in the ambivalent position of many liberal parents, not encouraging her children to have sexual encounters, but letting them know that she didn't disapprove.

Sally

Fifty-two. She has a son with schizophrenia and a daughter living abroad. She divorced when the children were young and has struggled financially and emotionally to bring them up as a single mother. Both children are still dependent on her.

My children were pretty offensive about men I brought home. I just thought life was work and kids. That nurturing period was not a sexual period for me, but I could also say that was to do with having been rejected and damaged by divorce.

I have several women friends of my own age who have expressed rampant sexual feelings about younger men, so we have compared notes. Some of them have actually consummated it. I think women are very close to their sons, and when they reach a stage when they feel relaxed with younger men because they feel old enough to be their mothers, then that's the dangerous point.

Put a woman with a young man around the same age as his mother, who is not his mother, but is also dealing with him because she is used to dealing with young people, I think it is a very volatile mixture. All the Greek myths have got a lot of truth in them.

It's also something about wanting something young and beautiful, and what is wrong with that! For a moment you can forget that you are getting older. To some extent you've got a power, you're deeply flattered that they fancy you and find you attractive.

Sex between the generations, particularly older woman – younger man, makes many people feel uncomfortable. But some younger men are clearly attracted to older women, without wanting to be mothered. While it is unlikely that women now in their eighties would have had a relationship with a much younger man, these are the new sorts of relationships that some modern women seem to be forming.

Maud

Seventy-eight. She is widowed. She has an open relationship with her children after a strong and happy marriage.

My daughter always says that she had an idyllic marriage. I used to think he was a very macho man, and I thought he treated her abominably but she was one of these adoring people, a real doormat.

My mother was a doormat, like many people in her generation, everything was for Daddy. I'm not at all, so maybe I am reacting against that. My daughter is a real homemaker, a real mother, she adored being pregnant. Her marriage nearly broke up at one point because she wanted a third baby. He wouldn't go near her, she refused to use any birth control. In the end she had her daughter.

Since my daughter has been a widow, she's got a man – I have a sin-in-law! They live in France, which is lovely but she is torn in two because she is a great mother character and none of her children is married. She has three children, the eldest is twenty-eight. I don't know, he had a long-lasting relationship with a girlfriend for about six years, she was Dutch. Since then he doesn't appear to have had any girlfriends at all, and I have wondered if he was gay.

The middle one is always falling in love and it is always disastrous and little Joy who is twenty-two, she had a relationship for four years and I could see the problem – her father died when she was eighteen and she had this boyfriend who was obviously her security and now it's broken up and I am very worried about her. The other grandchildren, Gordon is eighteen, I think he's frightened of sex and girls, I'm sorry for these youngsters.

Of my other children, the youngest has been happy, he's the stronger character in the family, which might be a reaction from me, because a lot of people would say that I was stronger than my husband. The elder boy has been married for twenty years. At one point, about three years ago the marriage nearly broke up. He's a social worker and he was having an affair, I don't think it had got to the sexual side, but his wife discovered and I felt so sorry for him, more than her. It's been a funny marriage really.

I don't envy the younger generation their freedom. I was lucky because I didn't have to worry about drugs or AIDS. I think Joy, the twenty-two year old, she must find it very difficult – everybody seems to get into bed with people, almost on the first date. It's the girl who suffers terrible dangers I think. And I feel very sorry for them, I'm very glad I didn't have to bring up my own children with all that.

The last word I would use to describe Maud is a doormat. She has lived her life as a strong, independent woman, even doing what she described as a Shirley Valentine on her husband when they were having difficulties in their marriage. The doormat phenomenon is rarer in younger women; financial independence has meant that women are no longer dependent for board and lodging on their husbands. It made me wonder how many women have put up with all sorts of abuse down the generations because there was no alternative.

Dot

Seventy. She has one daughter from her first disastrous marriage with a man she describes as a psychopath. She has seen a repeating pattern in her daughter's marriage and relationships. She has two grandchildren to whom she is very close.

My daughter has had a terribly damaged life. I knew she would make a disastrous marriage, which she duly did. She's not married to him now, she kept it very secret for twenty years, she just lived it and then after twenty years she rang to say she was leaving. I wasn't surprised, she did leave him for another man, but she didn't take the children and that really hurt me. But I can see why not and I understand they meant a lot to the father, so I propped the father up for two years until he could stand on his own feet. She still saw the children, she didn't leave them but walked out of the family home because there was no way he would ever allow her to go anywhere. The children were two and a half and eight, they are now nine and fifteen. The best thing is that from the very start I said to her that one day she would have to sort her life out and get therapy. She has now and she is sorting it out. This second relationship is almost as bad as the first, which again I could tell would have to happen! Yet again she is on the road, just leaving him now, and trying to look at herself as a person on her own.

I do envy the younger generation their freedom, not quite envy, I'm so pleased for them. I love my grand-daughter the way she can talk! The way she rang me up when she had her first period and said, 'Guess what!' It was a great celebration in our lives!

I think that is wonderful and I'm pleased that I told my daughter how hard sex was and told her to experience the joy of it, because we had been so restricted. My mother taking away my hands if ever they were seen in the wrong place and my sister and I being ticked off because we touched each other's bodies, and all these sad things that have made sex for me quite a handicap.

However much mothers might wish to protect their daughters from making mistakes, each generation has to follow its own path. All mothers can do is be there to pick up the pieces.

Chapter Nine

End thoughts

Joan

Fifty-two. She is celibate for religious reasons. She is the head of department in a local government planning office.

I don't think I have reached any wisdom or clarity after menopause, no I'd want to say no to that! It is a time of crisis, there is the feeling that time is running out, when you're young you had lots of goals and aspirations. You see the years slipping by and you realise that some things are just not going to be.

For me as a Christian, there are some things I would have loved to achieve, like going to darkest Africa, and I'm unlikely to do them now. I've been through some times of really having to say, 'No, I've just got to leave, I've just got to move on', and there's been a struggle to let go of some things that I've wanted to achieve and haven't. I must just move on and allow others to do some of those things. One gains a bit of perspective.

I'm basically happy and contented; celibacy has been a positive choice for me. One has to find one's own set of values, purpose in life and inner focus. There's lots of other ways you can give than within a marriage relationship. Happiness is a by-product and certainly not to be sought through another person; you have to find it in yourself.

Katherine

Fifty-three. She is coming to terms with changes in her marriage. Working after bringing up children has given her new perspectives.

I don't think menopause should affect you hugely. It is a step, another stage of your life and should be considered so. I don't think you should ignore it, or pretend it hasn't happened. You can't ignore these things, they are there and they are there to be built on and used in a very positive way. A lot of women like me, of a similar type, will think the same. I'm not exactly saying that I want to stay young forever, but I don't want it to be the reason for my cutting things down. I want it to be built on and I want to get more out of life because of it.

Marjorie

Seventy-six. She is divorced but still happy to be sexually active if the right opportunity comes along. Feisty and sure of her opinions, she laughs and swears like a trooper throughout our meeting. She is a woman full of life.

To someone coming up to menopause, I'd say 'Don't worry about it, don't think about it. When it comes, just get on with the rest of your life, you'll find that it will probably come very slightly, very gradually.' I've always been positive, I can't afford to be otherwise. If you're not positive, you're negative and then you go down the pan.

Annie

Fifty-six. Her perspective as a gay older woman is different. She feels an outsider on many fronts. She lives on her own.

I do envy the younger generation, I know it isn't easy for anybody whose sexuality isn't heterosexual because they've still got their family to cope with, and the people that they work with. But there are places they can go, there are books they can read, and if they're desperate, they can ring Gay Switchboard or Lesbian Line. My generation had nothing like that at all. I wasted years of my life being dreadfully, desperately lonely, much lonelier than I am now. I had nobody at all to talk to about my sexuality and that's a very lonely place to be.

Judith

Sixty-two. She is widowed with no children. She had a happy marriage and is prepared to have another go at a relationship but she is a little shy. She has a rich fantasy life.

I hope I'm wiser now, I surely must be, I've obviously gained knowledge throughout the years, along the way, about all sorts of things. I can see the mistakes that other people make and realise that there but for the grace of God go I. I hope I am clearer about things, although it often takes me quite a long time to decide what I want and what is best for me.

Do I look forward to the future? Not particularly for lots of reasons, the main one being that my mother is very elderly and I know that during the next ten years that I will lose her. Obviously other family and friends are getting older and I wonder what is in store for them as well as for me. I don't spend a lot of time worrying about it, it's going to happen, one accepts it when it does but I don't look forward with enjoyment.

I don't feel lonely, I suppose I do spend quite a bit of time on my own but that's mainly from choice, so I don't perhaps know what it's like to be really lonely.

More is made of the menopause than is necessary, although I do understand that a minority do suffer quite badly. Male doctors don't understand it very well, but I don't think it is something to be feared as much as some people think it is. I often think that the emotional aspect probably makes things worse rather than the actual physical symptoms. The fact that it's seen as the end of everything, whereas it certainly isn't! It isn't the end of sexuality, it's just the end of one's childbearing years. In fact, many people can be happier after menopause.

Clare

Fifty-six. She married twice and has children. Her second husband felt guilty on leaving his first wife and the sexual part of their marriage has not been a success. She is loyal, loving and affectionate. He is now seriously ill.

It's difficult, but I do think of when my husband is not going to be around, and I hope that I would meet someone. In a way his death would release me to meet someone else, someone who was not quite as complicated perhaps. I may again have a good physical relationship.

Caroline

Seventy-three. She has married three times, twice to the same man. Troubled marriages were not helped by being given LSD by a psychiatrist when they went for marriage guidance. She is worried that her children's problems may reflect her own difficulties.

I have become clearer and wiser about things, all experiences of your life teach you something as you go along. I know where I've made mistakes, done the wrong thing and what I have felt guilty and ashamed about, but I've worked through a lot of them. My children's troubles used to bother me more than they do now. I can often see the end of it for them whereas they can't. One learns.

My twin daughters are just beginning to go through menopause. The eldest is just about to start HRT. It seems strange to have daughters who are going through menopause, it doesn't make me feel older it makes me realise they are getting older! Menopause is something we all go through; it's really not something to be worried about, you can be just as attractive to your husband after as you were before. Don't worry about it or feel that life is coming to an end at all.

Madeleine

Seventy-three. She has had a long and happy marriage with a partner who fits. She radiates serenity and happiness. They have two children.

I think menopause varies so much, you can't say it's fine and you will get through it because I know that some women don't, but I must say once you're through the other side it's plain sailing!

I have more wisdom and clarity than when I was younger, I have a much wider span. But I don't think menopause has made any difference to the person I am.

Many women don't do what they want to do, indeed many women don't know what they want to do. They come to me and I say, 'Who are you?' and they say, 'I'm married to so and so', and I say, 'That's your wife role'. They say 'Well, I've got so many children', and I say, 'No, that's you as mother. Who are you?' And they have no idea. No self-worth, just dish rags. So that means they are living as mother and wife, as handmaiden. We have to teach young women to be their own person. They are not born to be married and to be mothers, they are people. Everyone has to have something they can look at, and say if it wasn't for me that wouldn't be there.

Jenny

Fifty-four. She is a happy, bright woman who used the crisis of menopause to sort out long-standing unhappiness. She is divorced and back on the dating game again. She has three children, two sons with learning difficulties and a younger daughter.

One does feel free after menopause. A lot of women think they're free from childbearing and haven't got to worry about contraceptives and getting pregnant any more. I was sterilised when I was forty-two, so that angle didn't affect me at all. I feel I'm a person now, worth something, and that has something to do with menopause. I don't have the awful monthly highs and lows, I'm stable. I really did feel I was not myself and now I feel I'm me.

Probably I'm what I've always striven to be now, what I was before I started having periods. I used to be calm and have a lot of spirit in me. The intervening years have been a blip – quite a blip! And now this is me! I like who I am for the first time in my life and that is thanks to the menopause. I used to be a great shouter but things don't seem to bother me the way they used to.

Florrie

Eighty-four. She is bundle of fun and energy. She married twice and has two children, now she has a live-in boyfriend in his sixties.

I've had a happy life all in all, I've done the things I wanted to do. Life has been more interesting since menopause, in some ways you feel more in charge of yourself.

I don't think I'm very wise, I think I'm very stupid really! I'm more informed I suppose, I've read widely. I don't think young people take any notice of us at all. But then I didn't take any notice of older people either when I was young.

I would recommend having children later on, I kept myself fairly decent for their sake. I'd got to keep young for them.

Mary

Forty-seven. Premature menopause because of a hysterectomy plunged her into deep depression. She has married twice, when she married her second husband she was still a virgin. She had three children, one died in infancy. She is trying to make sense of what has happened to her.

I feel I've come back on track, and I feel I'm wiser and clearer about all I have been through. I wish I could have been my own person more, enjoyed my life more, though not just so much from the sexual point of view. I sometimes think maybe I'm not as strong as I could be. I've never been on my own, I've always been in a relationship. I've never had to be my own person and fend for myself, I've always had someone there for me.

Dot

Seventy. She is a woman who came into her own at menopause. After a horrendous first marriage and countless affairs, she has now been happily married for twenty-five years. She has one daughter.

I know I have learnt more in the last ten years than in the whole of the rest of my life, and that each year I learn yet more. That little bit of wisdom that I am certain comes to you, comes to you out of looking at life completely differently. It's finally being honest with yourself but also there is so much to learn; about creation, what nature really is. I have blessed the fact that I have been given the time to learn all this, I wouldn't have understood half of what I now understand, I hadn't got time to study and think and just stand and stare. I see other people's needs completely differently, it makes me want to go on with the work I do.

Sally

Fifty-two. She is divorced and was left to bring up two children alone, and is bitter about the experience. She rediscovered her sexuality at menopause and seems to have a predilection for younger men, who are highly responsive to her.

Has menopause changed the way I feel about myself? I'm not cyclical any more, so that puts you on almost the same level as a man. It's not that I feel more manly, I feel like a warrior now, more powerful.

We get so much flak about it all. The post-menopausal bit is not what I expected, this feeling of power. I feel I could go into battle; I've gone back to the child I was.

I do finally think I can be who I want to be, and I do think the batty woman image is true to some extent and most people do run screaming away from it. If we do become ourselves, whatever that is, it is something that alarms people and I fear for my sisters when I see women of sixty-five going over the top.

I can be myself because I am beholden to no one now. I talk about twenty times more than I used to. I'm getting into my stride! I have the wisdom of time. I know that what I'm doing is what I should be doing. But I also feel more lonely sometimes and more vulnerable. I relish my solitude but I also sometimes feel very frightened of cancer, of dying, of being old alone, of getting more eccentric, of being persona non grata, the witch syndrome.

Conclusion

'I'm not cyclical any more, so that puts you on the same level as a man. I feel like a warrior now.' Listening to this woman talk about the cataclysmic changes she had been through at menopause, and how she had found her own strength and sexuality again after a lifetime of servicing her husband and then her children, showed that perhaps society is right to fear the unleashing power of such women. Many women reported 'losing' themselves in the demands of others. And that the empty nest syndrome, when the children finally left, although much feared, eventually gave them a chance to be themselves.

The experience of menopause could be broadly divided into three categories: those who found it very difficult physically; those who sailed through it; and those who had some symptoms, but were not unduly affected by it. But why do different women have different experiences and is it simply a question of hormones? It does seem that menopause in some way crystallises life experiences. That does not mean that if you have been a 'bad person' you have a terrible menopause, but rather that the easy or difficult parts of our lives seem to reappear at menopause. The women who had come to terms with their lives seemed, on the whole, to have had an easier time, while those who had had particularly difficult marriages or hellish childhoods went through a bad patch. Women who had suffered particularly badly from premenstrual tension suffered again when it came to menopause, but then felt wonderful relief to be through menopause and out the other side, free of periods at last.

The freedom of not having periods and the consequent enhancement of sex was mentioned by a lot of women. Many women also said they felt they had finally got back to the strong potential women they had been before periods started, something that had been lost in the intervening years taken up with fertility and childbearing. It was if they had lost their identity at puberty and picked it up again at menopause.

HRT seemed invaluable to some women: one woman was sure that she would have had to have been put away in a mental institution if HRT hadn't been available. She also sympathised with all those women in history who had been locked away because their behaviour was extravagant or simply unacceptable. But others didn't get on with it at all, many took it intermittently.

Women were more and more prepared to experiment with their health, with alternative medicine, for example, until they found something that worked for them. Sympathetic doctors were warmly praised, although drugs could also be depressing. The dry vagina syndrome worried many women, it directly affected how they felt about sex and made them feel less womanly. Public symptoms like hot flushes and sweats were universally dreaded, in part because they allowed others to categorise them as menopausal.

Several women had children in their forties and they seemed to feel that this helped them have an easier time at menopause, but that may have been because they were so preoccupied with bringing up young children that other symptoms and worries were disregarded.

Many women found that menopause was a rite of passage, helping them to confront horrors from the past that had lain dormant for many years. Child abuse, long-term depression and cruel and despotic parenting were all brought out into the open and worked through in therapy, allowing several women to come to a new point of balance that they had not felt for years.

Chapter 2 on marriage and long-term relationships threw up the most surprises. Older women are having all manner of relationships: live-in, live-out or live occasionally. Many had married more than once and two had remarried their first husbands.

Several stories stand out for me. The first is the youngest woman who knew nothing about sex, but thought that putting a ring on her finger would magically make things all right. She divorced her husband after thirteen months and was still a virgin when she married her second husband. The second is the woman who was treated with LSD for her marital problems. The pain and anguish of that experience caused the complete breakdown of their marriage. They both married again unhappily, and it was not until many years later that they finally found each other again and remarried. The pain of what now seems an unnecessary separation hung between us in that comfortable sitting room.

Then there was the woman whose husband asked her to go into the garden and get some birch twigs to beat him with, and who was not allowed a divorce by her family. And the woman who had stuck with a husband who had not been able to show her any affection, a strong warm woman who found warmth and affection in the next generation.

One woman realised during the course of our interview that she had never had a happy sexual relationship with the man she is married to and loves dearly. That stark thought had to be dealt with and we spent some time discussing what could be done about it.

Interviews often went on longer than planned, one could not leave such strong emotions and revelations or memories, happy or sad, abruptly after the allotted time.

There were happy marriages too, widows who spoke fondly of their partners even though the sex had not been wonderful, some who spoke wistfully of what might have been. And the couple who seemed blissfully happy, a current of electricity runnning between them, what was their secret? Respect, communication and a certain amount of good luck, plus a feeling that their relationship was meant to be.

The gay woman had run into all the ordinary problems when her relationship broke up, with the added pain that because she was not out of the closet, she could not share her grief with anyone. That was the biggest grief of all, and one that was still mourned.

Fidelity was a complicated chapter. From the women who had never looked at any one else to the woman who had an open marriage and had enjoyed herself very much. Many women thought about men, or fantasised about men they saw on buses or in supermarkets. When I see an older woman with a distant look, hanging by the cook chill cabinet, I'll no longer assume she has forgotten her glasses, I know she's probably looking at the dreamy young man in confectionery, like me!

They all had strong views on men, loved them or thought them a waste of space. One woman had discovered a taste for younger men at menopause and was delighted to find that they liked her too. She was fifty-two, but the woman of seventy-three who had recently finished an affair with a forty-four-year-old man still had a sparkle in her eye.

So what made some women give up on themselves, when others seemed ready for new relationships? Some of it had to do with self-image, but many women seemed to live or fight patterns which had been laid down by previous generations; one woman remembered not being allowed out late because of the fear of what the neighbours might think, which seemed to be the guiding light of her family's morality. She had allowed her children freedom so that they should not have to experience the same constraints.

Many saw celibacy as a relief, a breathing space before continuing with sex. The woman whose husband showed her no affection did not miss what had not been a very happy sexual life, though she longed for a cuddle at night. Many lived on good memories or were relieved it was all over. Some women found masturbation was enough.

And what effect did it have on me to listen to these stories? It made me question my own prejudices about older women, how we lump them all together despite the fact that there is as much difference between an eighty year old and a fifty year old as there is between a twenty year old and a fifty year old. I felt enormous respect for the way they had coped with disaster, tragedy or cruelty in their lives. But most of all it gave me hope for the future.

Biographies

Page references will enable you to follow each woman's path through the book.

Alice

Sixty. I see her at work where she is the boss of her own company in the Midlands. She describes herself as a walking disaster area as far as relationships are concerned. She resents having to work and not being taken care of by her husbands. She has married twice and is now living with the first husband again. She says that she attracts no-hopers. Clearly she is an efficient and capable woman. Yet she remains fixed in the idea that women should be taken care of, she dislikes her independence and the fact that she has always looked after the men in her life. She is a very sexual woman, loved having an affair with a musician and still enjoys flirting with men, although she would always wait for them to initiate in case of rejection. (See pages: 44, 85, 120, 151, 229, 238.)

Annie

Fifty-six. A gay woman who has found it hard to come to terms with her sexuality. She has even tried sleeping with men as a sort of medicine, she admits ruefully. Her sunny basement flat is full of affectionate cats. Dealing with lost relationships is difficult for heterosexual women; for older, closeted gay women it is even more painful. She feels caught in a trap of wanting a relationship but fearful of the pain and unsure of how to set about meeting someone again. Her self-image is low, she sees herself as enormously overweight, when she really looks pretty average in size. The packet of biscuits sits between us like an unspoken temptation. (See pages: 21, 71, 118, 169, 201, 226, 257.)

Brenda

Fifty-four. She sidles into the room rather shyly and is nervous of appearing boring – because she has had a happy marriage, great sex, loved being a mum and has never been tempted to stray. When she relaxes, she tells hilarious stories about her sexual escapades with her husband. She shines as she talks about him.

She is upset at the way society views women of her age, with lots to offer in the job market, and feels since she was made redundant that she has had to settle for a more menial job than she is worth. She is very frank and open, would like to become a counsellor, and is clearly a good listener as well as a good talker. She has lived in the same part of Norfolk for thirty years and has a clique of good women friends. She is shocked at the acceptance of menopause by some of them, their relief in giving up on themselves. She admits that when she went back to work after being a full-time mum, because her husband had been made redundant, she felt she had to develop a new Brenda, not the Brenda that they were all used to. (See pages: 46, 62, 115, 143, 199, 222.)

Caroline

Seventy-three. Archetypal Women's Institute, she is a capable practical woman. Her brother died in childhood of meningitis, and she feels this has made her a caring type in later life. Another brother was stillborn after her mother was hit in the abdomen with a cricket ball. This made her parents wildly over-protective of her. She was married happily with children until her husband had an affair. They went to a leading psychiatrist of the day and were both put on LSD for eighteen months which broke up their marriage and brought them both close to breaking point. She had terrible hallucinations about child abuse by her father, which she half suspects might be true. Then she married a concentration camp survivor with four teenage children. When he died, she eventually remarried her first husband and regrets their lost years when they could have had good counselling and made a go of it. She worries about the effect on her children's marriages, particularly one daughter who has married a man who has served time in prison for manslaughter – he caught someone in bed with his wife and took a carving knife to him. (See pages: 23, 80, 150, 176, 210, 243, 258.)

Clare

Fifty-six. Some women seem much younger than their years, and when Clare walks in wearing her slacks and sweater she looks ten years younger. She thinks before she answers and leaves gaps in the conversation as she faces what she has just said. She had married twice. Her second husband has always felt guilty about leaving his wife and children, and this has led to problems in their sex life. This was then compounded by his drink problem, and as a vicar in a small parish in Scotland, he had to leave and work abroad. She was left with the children and the feeling that the community was pointing at her as the family who had been in the local paper. Yet she describes her marriage as happy without much sex, even though her first marriage worked sexually. Her husband is now in bad health and she feels she cannot leave him. She has thought about the future and the possibility of other relationships. (See pages: 45, 77, 149, 173, 209, 229, 243, 258.)

Dot

Seventy. She has calm energy after a tempestuous life. She was abused by her father, who was mayor of the local town, so she was unable to tell anyone: who would have believed that such a good man would do such a thing? She fell in love at fourteen, a grand passion for a man who promised marriage and then married someone else. She ran off with another man and was forced to marry him, even though they had not slept together. On their wedding night he asked her to cut some birch twigs from the garden and beat him. She had a horrendous time with him. Eventually she got the courage to leave but was only allowed a separation, not a divorce, by her family for many years. After many affairs, she met another man who she has been happily married and faithful to for twenty-five years. She is frank and open about sex, has never had an orgasm, though she would like one before she dies! She almost had a breakdown at menopause and feels therapy after menopause has helped her come to terms with her past turmoil, and that she is now more her own person than she has ever been in her life. (See pages: 25, 105, 135, 157, 217, 234, 253, 261.)

Elizabeth

Seventy-seven. She walks with a stick. She has been married for many years to a man who can't show affection and who stopped having sex when she went through menopause, it seems almost symbolically. She had two children by a first husband who died and then more in her forties, which she believes meant she had an easier time at menopause because of having young children to look after. She speaks without bitterness about her husband, but feels pity that he has missed out on the warmth and affection she gets from other relationships with friends and her children and grandchildren. She has a fine sense of humour that shines through all the problems. She is glad that her children will not have to put up with what she has suffered. (See pages: 20, 74, 146, 172, 205, 227, 238.)

Evelyn

Fifty-six. She smoked and laughed throughout our interview. She is a social worker based in the north of England. She has a comfortable home in the country filled with dogs. She is smartly dressed with short hair. She has strong views on every subject, and is quite scathing about men. She has had a relationship with the same man for twenty years. They don't live together but see each other at weekends. He come over and digs the garden, they have dinner, watch Blind Date together, sleep together and then he goes home to his mother on Monday. It's an arrangement that seems to suit them both, a mix of companionship and independence. A warm, friendly, frank woman who comes from a large family. (See pages: 17, 148.)

Florrie

Eighty-four. She is recovering from a car accident, but has lost none of her vigour. She was brought up by repressive parents who were terrified of what the neighbours thought. Her mother took her to the doctor at seventeen when her period had not started, thinking that she had discovered some magical secret about sex, but worried that she might be pregnant! She married a much older man who was more like a brother than a husband and then, when he died, another man who knew about love-making and introduced her to the pleasures of a good sex life. She had children in her forties and an easy menopause. She reflects that had she not remarried, she might never have had good sex, and believes that a lot of women put up with things because they did not know any better. Now she has a live-in boyfriend in his sixties who is hopeless in bed, but she enjoys his company and would rather have a good night's sleep. She was determined that her children should not be restricted as she was. (See pages: 24, 93, 129, 180, 250, 260.)

Jenny

Fifty-four. Fashionably dressed in a peach jumper and slacks, she's vivacious and full of life. She always suffered from PMT and went through a horrendous menopause. Her marriage broke up during menopause, and she had to finally come to terms with the cruelty of her mother. She says she realised it was now or never, that she had to look at the anger she felt at her mother and took out on her husband. Therapy has restored her self-confidence, and she feels more herself than at any time in her life before. She has three children, two sons with learning difficulties and a fourteen-year-old daughter. She has started dating again and recounts hilarious and not so funny encounters. She has just met a man she thinks might turn into a relationship and is as nervous about it all as she was at twenty. (See pages: 36, 125, 153, 178, 196, 232, 249, 260.)

Joan

Fifty-two. A bright, smartly dressed woman comes to the door confounding my idea of what a spinster looks like. She has chosen to be celibate, she is an evangelical Christian and believes that sex should only take place within marriage and has not met the right man. We talk with amusement about Christian dating agencies. Her home is very feminine, with delicate colours and tapestries on walls and cushions. Celibacy has not been an easy decision for her; she struggled when she met a man she was attracted to, but she knew was not marriageable. She finds it hard to introduce the subject when having a relationship; how do you tell a man that you don't have sex? She holds down a senior post in local government planning and so has a lot of contact with men, which she enjoys. She tries hard to see men as people rather than men. (See pages: 51, 141, 163, 224, 255.)

Judith

Sixty-two. She had a happy marriage and is now widowed. She lives happily in a pretty village in the country. She has retired but has been asked back on a part-time basis by her firm, so she's pleased to feel still needed by them. She went through menopause after a hysterectomy, and felt it enhanced her sex life because it took all fear of pregnancy away. She has not been involved with anyone else since her husband died, but has a rich fantasy life, especially about younger men. (See pages: 49, 147, 207, 228, 242, 257.)

Katherine

Fifty-three. She looks younger and is fashionably dressed in a shortish skirt and matching cashmere jumper with a coral necklace. She likes to be able to 'pass' for a younger woman if she can. She realises during the course of our interview that she has never really had a very happy sex life with her husband, although she has always been faithful to him. She returned to work after bringing up a family and feels this has shifted the balance in their relationship; she is now the more powerful one. She has a thing about young men's necks on buses! (See pages: 49, 59, 119, 142, 161, 194, 221, 240, 256.)

Madeleine

Seventy-three. A calm smiling woman greets me at the door. She has the happiest marriage of the whole group, she and her husband radiate love and warmth. She had a miserable childhood – her father left and her mother tried to commit suicide and then died – which left her with problems showing affection, but her husband showed her how. They met at a dance and when he put his arms round her, they both felt that was it, and visibly still do. She believes the secret of a good marriage is respect and communication and luck – they were meant to be together. (See pages: 42, 88, 122, 152, 211, 230, 246, 259.)

Marjorie

Seventy-six. She opened the door to me in a black leather trouser suit and it was all downhill from there! Coffee is made and generously laced with brandy. Her beloved dogs surround her in her terraced suburban house in Wales. Feisty and with strong views, she spends some time discussing current politics and she voices her disgust at the government. She has recently been on marches to protect the environment. The youngsters tried to protect her from the police until they realised she could outwalk and outshout them all, and any young policeman who dared to be cheeky to her would not live long. (See pages: 15, 65, 117, 144, 168, 192, 256.)

Mary

The youngest woman at forty-seven. She had a hysterectomy at forty-five, which plunged her into a terrifying menopause with all the worst symptoms exaggerated and accelerated – panic attacks, loss of memory, sweats, flushes, dry vagina, terrible depression. She feels she would have had to be put in a mental home if HRT had not been available. She had already suffered a lot of trauma. She married at twenty, believing that it would magically make everything work, only to divorce thirteen months later, still a virgin. She married a widower with three children and then lost a twin baby. She feels she is just beginning to see daylight. I was shocked by her youth when I met her, I assumed she must be the daughter of the woman I had come to see. (See pages: 28, 95, 130, 215, 261.)

Maud

Seventy-eight. She is a smartly dressed, bright woman who was widowed after a long and happy marriage. She felt there were two important turning points in her marriage: when he tried to physically restrain her early on, she left the house for two days, until he came to get her and apologise; and when he became so wrapped up in his business that he stopped noticing her, she did a Shirley Valentine and took herself off to Tenerife until he did take notice. She prefers intellectual men and feels that women worry about her effect on their husbands because she is bubbly and bright. She has no desire for a man now, and finds masturbation sufficient, although she would like a dinner companion and someone to go on holiday with. (See pages: 27, 100, 132, 136, 156, 186, 216, 234, 252, 262.)

Mavis

Seventy-three. She is a no-nonsense bundle of energy who lives in a sunny council flat with stunning views over the city. Widowed ten years ago after a happy marriage, she believes the secret of her youthful looks, health and happiness to be a good sex life. It doesn't matter if you no longer have one, as long as you did at some time! She sailed through menopause except that all her hair fell out. It has now grown back and is beautifully coiffed. She would not dream of going out of the house without looking smart and with make-up on, and believes young people should make more effort. She recently finished an affair with a forty-four-year-old man which she describes as delightful. (See pages: 40, 91, 124, 140, 170, 213, 231, 248.)

Rose

Eighty-four. Meeting Rose was like shaking hands with history. She has lived in the same area of London all her life. She grew up in poverty and has struggled all her life. She went out cleaning offices while bringing up her children and nursing an invalid husband. She is not bitter but is politicised by her life, and glad that her children and grandchildren have better lives. She is keen on her family, there are photos all round the flat. She is proud that she washed her own walls down last year, though she hasn't got round to it yet this year. She campaigns for rights for the elderly. We sit in her kitchen where it is warmer and drink lots of coffee. She speaks frankly about the ignorance of sex in her generation and rather wistfully of what might have been. She gives me a pot of excellent homemade marmalade and kisses me warmly on the cheek as I'm leaving. (See pages: 18, 69, 121, 175, 201, 225, 241.)

Sally

Fifty-two. She has come into her own since menopause, and now feels like a warrior. She brought up two children on her own after a divorce. She feels bitter that motherhood stifled her sexuality, which she is only beginning to express again with younger men. An artist, she has a fine sense of humour and laughs at herself and her adventures. She has had terrible physical symptoms, bleeding so bad that she had to wear pads, and carry a towel round with her to sit on other people's furniture. She feels she is now the woman she potentially was before her periods started and is making up for lost time. (See pages: 33, 155, 181, 214, 232, 251, 263.)